THE POWER OF THE RAYS

The Science of Colour-Healing

By

S. G. J. OUSELEY

Author of Colour Meditations, Science of the Aura, *etc.*

L. N. FOWLER & CO. LTD.

1201-1203 HIGH ROAD, CHADWELL HEATH,
ROMFORD, ESSEX RM6 4DH

First Edition March 1951
First Impression December 1954
Second Impression March 1957
Third Impression January 1961
Fourth Impression January 1963
Fifth Impression July 1967
Sixth Impression January 1969
Seventh Impression December 1970
Eighth Impression November 1972
Ninth Impression January 1975
Tenth Impression May 1976
Eleventh Impression July 1981
Twelfth Impression May 1983
Thirteenth Impression September 1986

0 8524 3063 9

Publishers Note

The Cosmic Colour Fellowship
was closed on the death of the
founder Mr. S. G. J. Ouseley.

Printed and bound in Great Britain by A. Wheaton & Co. Ltd, Exeter

CONTENTS

FOREWORD

THE author is confident that this little volume will be found of practical value to all people who are engaged in, or who aspire to, the great work of Healing.

The favourable reception accorded to the writer's previous book on Colour, i.e. *Colour Meditations*, gives rise to the hope that the new work will be equally well received.

In a little-known subject such as Colour there is always the danger for enthusiastic minds to be carried away by speculation and theory, and if that tendency is not kept checked much harm may be done to the whole cause of occult scientific research.

The author earnestly hopes that the care he has taken to deal with facts that are substantiated rather than fantasies will be apparent to the candid reader. It is hoped that the teachings set out in this volume will radiate into the minds and hearts of all who study them a light and an influence that will powerfully provide the ideal of Radiant Health and Service.

Chapter 1

COLOUR IS A CURATIVE POWER

THERE is every reason to believe that Chromotherapy or the use of Colour in the treatment of disease may at some period not far distant take its place as a recognised science. It cannot be denied that the cures obtained by the agencies of Colour and Mind stand out as living witnesses of the power that is wielded by them.

It is unfortunate that the general dearth of literature and the high prices charged for text-books and courses on Colour have resulted in a widespread lack of knowledge concerning this vital subject.

Of recent years we have heard much of sun baths, ray treatment, electricity, radiant heat and what not, and it is gradually becoming recognised that the finer and especially the etheric forces of Nature are of more avail than the raw, crude mineral and material substances, which are now often only used by intelligent physicians simply because their patients would think it peculiar if they did not prescribe drugs and bottles of medicine.

The Light cure is Nature's own. Animals bask in the glorious rays of the solar orb on which the entire life of this planet depends, and the Italians have a proverb, *Dove il sole non entra, entra il dottore*. ("Where the sun does not enter, the doctor does.")

Many years ago the famous American Colour scientist, Dr. E. Babbitt, patented an intricate apparatus which he termed the *Chromolume*, designed to transmit the sun's rays through coloured glass. It was rather cumbersome and in any case could not be applied very successfully in

a climate like ours, depending as it did on unlimited
sunshine.   More recently there have been evolved a
number of Colour Lamps using electric lighting and these
can be employed quite successfully in a wide variety of
cases.   The Cosmic Colour Fellowship will be pleased to
supply readers with details of such Colour Lamps which
are reasonably priced.

To comprehend the principles of Colour Therapy
completely would take more space than can be given here,
but the various aspects of the subject are fully treated
by Dr. Babbitt in his monumental work, *The Principles
of Light and Colour* (now out of print).

It is perhaps sufficient for the ordinary reader and
healer to understand the main points of the theory and
then to pass on to their practical application.

The source of all terrestrial life—the Sun—contains
within it practically everything of which the earth—and
its inhabitants—are composed, and if there be any
potency in drugs that potency is intensified by coming
direct from this centre of Life and Force.   It is therefore
not surprising to find that the colours which the Spectroscope reveals are indicative of various metals and gases
given off in the form of others varying in intensity and
quality, some of these colours being termed *heat* or *thermal*
colours, and the others *cold* or *electric*.   As Babbitt
observes, " The trinity of colours, red, yellow and blue,
is represented in the three great elements of hydrogen,
carbon and oxygen which constitute so much of the world,
including the whole of a large portion of the sugars, gums,
starches, ethers, alcohol, many acids, and much of the
substance of the vegetable world."

Coloured glass hinders the passing through of certain
rays and when these are precluded interesting results are
effected.   Experiments have shown that plants grown

under red glass shoot up four times more quickly than in ordinary sunlight, and that slower growth occurs under green or blue glass. The reason for this, of course, is that Red is the Life Ray: it stimulates vitality, whereas Blue and Green do not stimulate but slow down.

As will be seen later, the Red Ray is excellent in treating all debility conditions, and the Blue and Green Rays act as sedatives and relieve excitement and inflammation.

It is well known that in Nature heat associates itself with Red. Fire and Anger is of this colour: so, too, are the capsicum, cloves, musk, balsam of Peru and other plants used as drugs, the tints varying from bright red to dark brown. In diseases heat is expressed by redness, as in inflammation, fevers, etc. In the emotions, people turn red with passion and anger. The colour itself suggests warmth and hence it is a favourite tint in cold weather and cold rooms. Blue is usually associated with lack of warmth: we describe people as being blue with cold. Snow and ice have a bluish tint and drugs which are employed to relieve inflammation, or as astringents, nervines, etc., are frequently blue in colour. Broadly speaking, Chromotherapy is based upon these natural correspondences and the results achieved amply support this theory.

Disease is a want of harmony in the system, or in other words a want of colour and the object is to restore or supply this colour-deficiency.

Observation shows that people of certain complexion are predisposed to a definite type of disease, and the practised eye of a healer detects at once the class of disease to which a man is liable.

Following on the heels of Dr. Babbitt, Dr. Ponza, Dr. Hale, Dr. Pancoast, General Pleasanton in the West, we find enthusiastic Colour Healers in India and the East, including Jwala Prasad Jha, who devoted many years to the practice of the Science and successfully combated the dreadful scourge, the plague, in Bombay.

The two most important colours employed in Chromotherapy are *red* and *blue*. Long standing and complicated diseases require modifications of these, as will be explained later. As a general rule, Red should be used where there is a lack of vitality, where there is emaciation, and where the hands and face assume a blue tinge in cold weather, also in deficient nutrition, dormant conditions, depression, cold inflammations, paralysis.

Blue is applied to all conditions where inflammation is present (except cold as above stated), inward bleeding, nervous conditions—it is cooling, sedative, astringent, and healing generally.

Green is useful combined with Blue or Red, and Yellow is a brain and nerve stimulant, also emetic and laxative. The Orange Ray (a mixture of Red and Yellow) is powerful in cold, sluggish or chronic conditions. Other mixtures of Colours are useful in their place, and will be mentioned later.

As to the apparatus required, a Colour Lamp to be effective should consist of seven plates or slides, viz. :— Red, Orange, Yellow, Green, Blue, Indigo, Violet or Purple.

In addition to the Coloured Lights great assistance is obtained by using water that has been charged by the Colour Rays, to be used internally or in fomenting or bathing with. For this purpose, any glass bottle or tumbler may be used. Place them with a little water in the Colour Rays or in the sunlight a few minutes and administer in small doses.

Clothing exposed to the Rays becomes charged with

special beneficial effects according to the colour. Further particulars about Colour Treatments will be found in the author's book *Colour Meditations*, obtainable at Fowler's.

Food as well as water is capable of transmitting the potency of the rays if exposed a short time to them, and the taste is in no way interfered with.

CHAPTER 2

COLOUR-HEALING THEORY AND PRACTICE

CHROMOTHERAPY, or Colour Healing, is the treatment of diseased conditions of Mind and Body by the use of various Colour-Rays. Concisely speaking, there are two main types of healing, viz. : contact healing and absent healing.

In Contact healing use is made, either consciously by the operator or under special direction, of the " ultra " or Cosmic Colour Rays blended with the natural colours of the physical solar spectrum. Absent treatment is conducted by means of meditation and concentration, the absent patient having in his possession a small piece of some material vitalised by the healer and symbolising by its colour the basic healing ray.

The principle at the back of Colour Healing is the vibrational increase of the physical and etheric cells with the aid of a Colour Ray Projector. The centres or avenues through which the ray-force enters are the psychic inlets known as the chakras (Hindu—" Wheels or centres of force "), of which there are seven main ones. In its higher vibratory state, the physical body becomes more sensitive and receptive to the healing force which flows through the healer via the etheric and subtle bodies— thus the disharmony is corrected.

In Contact Healing, the healer concentrates his mind or eye upon the Aura of the patient (some healers see objectively with the eye, others see subjectively with the mind). The diseased condition or organ will be seen

14

reflected in the Aura at a point nearest to the actual counterpart in the physical body. The healing ray is directed at the appropriate chakram or inlet which is regarded as the patient's centre of polarisation. If Auric clairvoyance is not developed or possessed by the healer, the latter passes his right hand over the patient's body, gently and softly, until he comes to some part where a vibration of the finger tips or slight oscillation of the finger manifests the seat of the disease.

The appropriate colour ray is then sensed and the projector is focused upon the glandular centre requiring re-charging.

A secondary asset in the healing process is a glass of drinking water, which is charged by being held in the healer's hand for five minutes. The patient should drink the water very slowly, at the same time absorbing the " power " mentally. It is not unusual for the patient to declare that the water has a slightly alkaline taste.

A further aid in the treatment is Colour Massage. The healer having first washed his hands in tepid water, proceeds to bathe them for from three to five minutes in the full rays of the Colour lamp. They are then rubbed briskly together and massage is then given for ten to fifteen minutes. It is important to realise that Colour, like other forces and energies in nature, is either positive and negative in its effect—either beneficial or harmful. It is of the utmost importance that we should cultivate the right colour vibrations in and around our bodies and surroundings. A great deal of the discord and incompatibility between members of families and groups of people closely associated together is caused by cross-vibrations which are aroused by the predominance of some one or more inharmonious colours within some personal aura or environment.

When the predominating colour vibration or auric emanation of any two individuals in close proximity to each other are not in harmony there is no possible chance for peace or mutual understanding to exist between these persons unless they can neutralise the inharmonious vibrations by manifesting some other colour vibration which will blend with the former.

By the study and examination of the aura of a person it can be determined easily what colour vibrations the subject is most deficient in and what colours should be worn constantly on the body in some form. The necessary colour must contact as nearly as possible the centre of the body requiring recharging and must be worn until the revitalising vibrations have induced the new conditions or strengthened the centres. These cross vibrations are largely responsible for " nerviness " and can never cure ill-health. Both the psychological and the biological properties of the different colours have to be understood and adapted to suit particular individuals. For example, it would not only be unwise but positively harmful for the average Westerner or European to wear the yellow robe or turban of the Oriental yogi. Only in comparatively few cases could the colour yellow be beneficially worn continuously by a native of Europe or America. The vibrations of Red, Blue, Green are more generally necessary in the West.

The powerful effects of colour vibrations have been ascertained by many scientists. In her book on *Spectrobiology* Maria de Charpowichi writes : " In my laboratory work I have exposed microscopic cells of various organisms such as Algae, Infusoria, Yeast, Bacteria to either direct or diffused sunlight as well as to various types of artificial illumination through colour filters of various wave-lengths. The specimens are placed in individual dishes covered with coloured glass or gelatine transmitting only a selected range of light. Ultimate results have proved that each colour has a specific function to perform in the development of normal life and that this life-promoting, biological potency is contained within a particular range of intensity, correlated to certain elements contained within the protoplasm (Basic Life-substance) and which under the stimuli of that colour become actively potent."

Those who are familiar with the occult teaching of the sevenfold division of all matter force and consciousness will understand the statement that the seat of any disease is in the etheric centre of the organ affected. Basically speaking, the energy which is emanated from the " white " ray of undifferentiated light becomes differentiated as Colour on the etheric plane. This plane or vital sphere, as it more correctly is, acts as a screen or sensitised plate which receives and transmits the energy as colour within itself. As individual groupings of the different aspects of colour, these groups are reflected in the auric sphere of man and thence to the etheric body whence they become the substratum of the organs and different desires of the physical man. While these groups all have some one predominating colour, they contain potentially all other colours, and these colour vibrations being subject to the energy of Mind and Will are subject to change in degrees of shade and intensity, according to the nature and intensity of the light forces operating upon or within the groupings. The student may here feel inclined to ask— by what process does disease manifest itself ? Of old we have been told that *diseases are manacles forged by the mind of man.* How are these *manacles* forged ? Take, for example, the case of a victim of consumption. At some stage of his existence he first lays a line of thought, the basic subject of which is intimately connected with one astral centre of a physical organ.

This line of thought will probably be associated with some form of harmful self-indulgence and if this wrong activity is more intimately connected with a breath centre, the soil or habitat suitable for the disease elementals of tuberculosis will be created in the throat or lungs. These disease elementals are always with us but they can do no harm until a suitable environment is created for them. Embodied in the bacillus they will at once commence to destroy the tissue forming the organ. As a necessary environment can only be created by self-indulgence the conditions for recovery can only be created by sacrifice. The centre—the colour—must be purified so that it will no longer afford nourishment for the tubercular bacilli— the "devourers." This is achieved by a positive mental attitude towards health and also by the cessation of these appetites or habits of self-indulgence which originally caused the disease. It is also of importance to tune in the physical body wit!: the healing vibrations of nature.

The Colour and Light method of treating disease is based on true scientific values—the effect of the majority of ordinary methods is to drive the disease from one plane or organ to another.

The view has at times been put forward that Light or Colour cannot produce healing effects unless a vast volume or quantity is used. This is quite erroneous. It is not the amount or intensity but the quality of light that produces healing. Increasing or augmenting the quantity does not make any appreciable difference as the general reactions take effect only after a definite period. This is due to the Law of Periodicity and the fact that the protoplasmic impulses and reactions recur at definite intervals— according to a fixed rhythmic pattern.

Rhythm is the basic expression of all physiological and subconscious mental functions.

The whole organism performs various automatic rhythmic actions such as the heart beat, the breathing process, the blood circulation ; so each individual cell performs cyclic processes rhythmically at definite intervals.

In view of these facts we would impress on students the importance of time-periods in Colour Therapy—if the exposure is wrongly timed there is the danger of harm done even though the Colour Ray used is the correct one. The practical point to remember is that the repeated and continuous use of the appropriate colour vibrations is much more effective than a brief exposure to any form of intense radiation.

Intense or powerful illumination will produce more heat-vibrations but not necessarily greater healing power.

The best length of time for a Colour or Ray Treatment is thirty minutes or a little less.

The practical application of Colour to the human body falls into two divisions, viz. :—

(1) General diffusion and (2) Local concentration.

In treatment by general diffusion the method consists in focusing the light rays all on the body, with special reference to the back. It is excellent as a general tonic for recharging the tired cells with new vitality. The patient should either sit or lie down in a relaxed position, stripped to the waist, and should be wholly immersed in the light for thirty minutes.

Should the treatment be extended to one hour it is advisable for the patient to be in a lying position.

The local concentration, the light-vibration, is focused on the affected area only. The same colour filters are used, the colour, of course, being of the requisite ray for combating the specified disease. An exposure of from fifteen to twenty minutes is the normal procedure, the local treatment then being followed by a general diffusion of thirty minutes.

The great value of chromotherapy as a remedial agent lies in the penetrative power of light. Light and colour have a direct action on the protoplasm of the body—the speed and power of the chemical and other reactions depend upon the biological state of the organism.

Radiation is still a subject little understood by scientists and the penetrating properties of certain cosmic rays are even more marvellous than those of light.

Exactly how light penetrates or influences the body is not easy to comprehend. Some scientists are of the opinion that the penetration is simply a process of osmosis (permeation of the cells). But the generally accepted view is that light and colour penetrate and influence the body activity by arousing sympathetic vibrations within the organism. In other words Light and Colour work according to the Law of Attraction.

As most students are already aware, all physical bodies are components of electro-magnetic points of energy or elements in a refined state of rarefication. Concisely speaking, health is the condition of perfect equilibrium between these elements—but that equilibrium is only maintained as long as there is perfect rhythm and harmony throughout the organism.

In studying the nature of light it is important to remember that all radiations emitted from a luminous body travel through space in perfect rhythmic vibrations in the form of waves. The point or distance from crest to crest of these vibratory waves is called their wave-length and their " beat " or rate of vibration is known as their frequency. The wave-lengths of various colours differ greatly. For instance, Violet light consists of very short waves, while Red light consists of much longer ones.

As a wave or light is projected through space it creates a certain rhythm—an harmonious vibration of etheric matter. When light and colour strike a surface the homogeneous particles are thrown into sympathetic vibrations with the incoming current corresponding to the frequency of the stimulating ray. As a result the organism is revitalised or recharged. If, however, the particles within the body are non-conductive or an opposite rate of vibration or if the intensity and power of the incoming current is stronger than the normal resistance rate of the body, then an abnormal reaction will occur which may produce serious harm or damage. It is extremely important to know the correct nature of the light or colour we intend using—its quality, quantity and intensity. The whole basis of Colour healing consists in causing certain molecular reactions in the organs through the medium of the rays. Light, it should always be remembered, is not a force or energy outside us—light enters into the centre of every cell, nerve and tissue of our bodies. Nature has given us this wonderful form of energy which is the basis of life, to sustain our minds and bodies alike in perfect health.

In conclusion, it may be of interest to mention an important aspect of healing through the Aura. The following statement occurred in an address by Laughing Waters, the spirit guide of Ellen Warren:

" It is important that you should live in harmony with the colours in your own aura, in connection with your own surroundings. You may say, perhaps, that a certain colour does not suit you ; that is because deep within your own aura there is the consciousness that this colour is not in harmony with you. Many of you are healers. If you come to someone who is sick your own guides and helpers immediately come close to you and begin to work upon your own aura. They enhance the colours which are needed in your aura to be given to the sick person. They bring great power to you. Perhaps some of you have felt it as a tingling in your finger tips. What is happening is that those of spirit, working upon the colour vibration, are bringing to your particular aura that colour which is needed for the said person. When you begin to make your little prayer, the patient becomes tranquil and quiet, and the vibrations of colour in your own aura begin to permeate the person and replenish the faded colours where they are needed in the aura of the sick one."

(See *Psychic News* No. 796.)

Chapter 3

THE HUMAN AURA

In the human organism the manifestation of Colour is based upon the sevenfold nature of Man.

Man is a septenary being. Orthodox writers speak of Man as body, soul and spirit. This is a convenient and condensed classification of the main principles of Man ; in the more detailed and accurate analysis of esoteric science Man is considered in seven aspects. This sevenfold division is in agreement with the great septenary principles of nature.

In the esoteric analysis of the manifold phenomena of life, occultists see seven main states of being or levels of consciousness.

Psychology shows that our mental activity is not limited to one *conscious* plane—there is a subconscious and super-conscious region of the mind. Indeed our conscious life is in reality a *reflection* of our deeper interior mental and spiritual conditions.

Occult science classifies the phenomena of mental and soul-life within the following basis :—

1. Physical-Etheric plane
2. Astral plane
3. Lower Mental plane
4. Higher Mental plane
5. Spiritual-Causal plane
6. Intuitional plane
7. Divine or Absolute plane

The seven aspects of man as defined above are not separative states distinct from one another, but are the currents of thought and feeling flowing in the ocean of consciousness—they infiltrate and overlap.

Man is thus evolving seven principles or aspects which go to make up his complete being—four of which are more directly concerned with ordinary mundane existence —the physical, the etheric, the astral, the mental—whilst the remaining three appertain to the spiritual.

Before beginning a study of the Colour-aspects of life, it is of the utmost importance that the student should understand the composition and function of the human *Aura.**

The Aura is the expression of the *real man*, a manifestation of the state and degree of his sevenfold nature. It is the sum-total of his forces and emotions—physical, etheric, astral, mental and spiritual—of the individual. Concisely speaking, it is a subtle, super-physical emanation surrounding a person in the form of a luminous mist or cloud.

The auric emanation is the essence of a man's life—it reveals his character, emotional nature, mental calibre, state of health and spiritual development.

Everything in nature generates its own Aura, atmosphere or magnetism. In human beings the extent and strength of the Aura varies considerably—so also does its configuration. Apart from clairvoyant investigation the facts concerning the Aura are borne out by the recent experiments of scientific investigators in this field.

The researches of Dr. Kilner and his colleagues have done much in this direction. The accidental " discovery " of Professor A. W. Goodspeed of the Randal Morgan Laboratory of Physics at the University of Pennsylvania, that rays of light emanate naturally from the human body and that these rays are visible to the eyes of some of the

* See *The Science of the Aura*, by S. G. J. Ouseley.

lower animals, merely corroborates a truth that has been known to occultists for centuries.

The rays of light in the human atmosphere, though invisible to the unassisted human eye, are perfectly visible to clairvoyants, and by the aid of intricate lamps and chemicalised screens ordinary investigators can map out their area and conformation. Tests have shown that the Aura is capable of being electrified, and experiments with argon-filled lamps placed within the " sphere of influence " have caused the Aura to light up.

The early Church made an attempt to popularise the idea of the Aura by depicting a circular-shaped cloud of a golden colour around the head of the saints. The Aura, however, is not restricted to any particular part of the body.

The auric emanation consists of seven distinct units or waves of light encircling the subject in an oval shaped conformation. Its composition, definiteness and extent will depend on the measure of the subject's progress and evolution. In some cases it will extend a few inches only, in other cases such as the Aura of an initiate or seer, the extent may be several feet.

The key to an understanding of the Aura is to be found in the nature of man.

We have seen that man is a septenary being evolving along seven planes of life—the physical, etheric, astral, lower mental, higher mental, and three spiritual planes. All these aspects of consciousness manifest in the Aura.

The seven-fold Aura is thus the true guide to a man's soul and character.

The student of Colour Science will need to fix the main principles of the Aura carefully in his mind.

First Aura. Emanating from the physical body and enveloping it in a cloud-shaped conformation is the first or *health* Aura. It is compounded of the physical and etheric forces in man's being and is based on a centre in the spine. The vital solar force (life energy) is absorbed by the etheric body and reflected in the health aura as a pale reddish colour. In health the vital force radiates in straight regular lines in every direction from the periphery of the body. In cases of disease or ill-health the radiations are seen to droop, bend or crumble, at points where the lack of solar force is causing the state of inharmony. In good health the force of these auric emanations is sufficient to protect the physical body from inimical germs and bacteria.

Illness in its multitudinous forms and conditions arises when the etheric radiations are weak or feeble—the common phase " being run down " aptly expresses the drooping radiations.

Second Aura. This Aura emanates from the astral or emotional centre in the spleen and encircles the astral body, extending for a distance varying from 12 to 18 in. Its strength and colour depend entirely on the individual with whom it is connected. The colours vary with the nature of the man—these astral colours are of an almost infinite variety. With every change of thought, emotion, desire and feeling, there is a corresponding change in the astral Aura. The astral body is the vehicle or mode of expression of the emotional and passional nature.

It changes its colour continually as it vibrates to the motions of thought.

When the astral Aura is in harmony with the other parts of man's being it shines forth bright and luminous—a glorious sight. When there is disharmony or any un-balance in the emotional nature, the Aura reveals dark spots, dull and murky patches. Thus the astral Aura is a true guide to the psychological condition.

Third Aura. There are two aspects or vehicles of mind —the lower objective mind, and the higher or subjective. In the one sphere of mind man reasons and acts in accordance with his degree of knowledge and intelligence ; in the other, the subjective mind, he makes use of higher forces and faculties according to his degree of development.

The twin mind-aspects are reflected in the third and fourth Auras.

The lower mental Aura reflects the essence of man's natural and intellectual energies. Its strength and manifestation depend upon the degree of mental organisation and the way in which the mental attributes and qualities are developed. It is oval, egg-like in outline, emitting a radiant pale yellow colour as it develops.

It increases, in size and activity, incarnation after incarnation, with the growth and development of man himself.

In the well-balanced, intelligent and mentally-alive individual, the Aura is a resplendent, shiny picture. When the mental consciousness is evil, corrupt or perverted, the thoughts are reflected in the Aura and cause dark spots, defamed and grotesque *forms*, and the colours become transformed into various tones and hues which have a definite meaning.

Fourth Aura. This is an emanation of the higher mind —the soul principle. It is a reflection of our higher mental activities. *Its colour tone is Green.* It is the realm of the Cosmic consciousness and soul-experience far transcending the limited region of the objective mind. The higher centres of inspiration and intuition have their source in the subjective (abstract) mind. It is the field of *true* music, poetry and art in the highest sense, and their essence is out-pictured in the fourth Aura.

The Colour tone of this Aura is basically Green, although some of the highest cosmic colours are reflected in it, transforming it into an object of extraordinary beauty.

The manifestation of thought through the medium of colour and also sound is a form of infra-mundane symbology of which the ordinary mind is not usually aware. Colour-language has been spoken of as the " language of the gods." It is not to be implied that the mind " thinks " a colour, as a sound, or a form—it thinks a thought a subtle and complex vibration, which becomes manifested in these respective modes according to the vibration set up.

The substance of the mental realm is continuously being thrown into vibration from which ensue colours, sounds and forms.

The mental Aura grows and expands by thought-force. The bright radiating colours in the mental Aura are produced by the exercise of our mental faculties, artistic powers and higher emotions. We are literally colouring our Auras hour by hour and day by day. Nothing *colours* the Aura more than habitual thought. If your intellectual powers are dormant—if you are like a passive machine instead of an active, vital force, your mental Aura is dimmed and invisible.

The very moment you focus your mind upon developing the colours in your Aura you begin to evolve and advance and your soul-experience will grow richer.

Fifth Aura. Interpenetrating the realms of the etheric, astral and mental is the spiritual—the true cause of the strange and perplexing phenomena of life. The fifth Aura manifests the essence of the spirit, or causal body. According to occult science, all effects and conditions in the lower planes of life are manifestations or results of the forces within the spiritual or causal body.

This body is the form-aspect of the individual—it is the epitome of the soul's life-history. It acts as the receiving station of all the activity sent out by the lower nature, and indelibly records every impression. The lower Auras are vitally affected by the state of the causal body.

The fifth Aura is the point of union between the cosmic and the individual. It is like a delicate band marking where the individual begins his separate life and it persists from one incarnation to another through the whole period of human evolution. In the *Vedas* it is called the " thread-self," the re-incarnationary ego. No other particle of man's being can outline it.

The causal Aura is hardly perceptible in most people— only in advanced souls is it clearly visible as the true presentation of the man. The radiance then transcends anything earthly—its colours are exquisite and delicate, showing sub-tones that are indescribable as they are totally different from the earthly colour spectrum. Its dominant colour is represented to our vision by certain ethereal shades of blue.

Sixth and Seventh Auras. These higher Auras belong rather to the Cosmic aspects in man than to any of the human principles. They blend together in an effulgence of brilliant light at the outer edge of the Aura, and are rarely seen except around the bodies of initiates and masters.

The highest vibration of all, the White light, is not generated by the individual ; but is projected or transmitted to the Aura from the supreme Cosmic Source. All other colours emanate from within man's being.

The White light is projected with the seven auric centres, or chakras, where it is absorbed.

The beams of White light play a fundamental part in the function and well-being of our inner-bodies. When this divine light flows harmoniously into the interior centres, our condition is rendered healthy and harmonious. When there is a stoppage or obstruction the opposite state prevails. For example, suppose the White light does not properly reach our etheric body—this indicates that some organ or gland is not functioning correctly.

The point where the White beam stops is the point where some negative or faulty conditions exist creating a definite " block."

Let us suppose the White beam stops at a point in the second Aura ; this would indicate a *wrong* condition in the astral (emotional) side of man's nature. The fault is transmitted to the lower White and the effect is manifested in the etheric centre and the physical body. The cause is in the astral body, but the ultimate effect is experienced in the physical in the form of some diseased state or complaint. It should be remembered that the law " as above, so below " applies very markedly in the science of colour and auric intuition as elsewhere in nature. The higher bodies affect the lower, but not vice versa.

From the foregoing it will be understood that the Aura is a living map, as it were, of a man's life—a colour chart of his mind and soul, a key to his character, his personality and potentialities as well as his faults and complexes. Auric analysis is much more subtle and penetrating than psycho-analysis, and also much more comprehensive as it deals with all the planes of human consciousness.

CHAPTER 4

THE PHYSICAL BODY

THE physical body—the temple of flesh in which the spirit of man dwells for a time—consists of two parts, viz. : (1) a visible part and (2) an invisible part.

To occult students the first part is known as the dense or corporeal body and the second part is termed the etheric double or the vital-body. They are correctly classed together as they both function on the physical plane, are both composed of physical matter and are cast off by the human spirit at death and disintegrate together.

These dual principles of the physical nature both belong to the lower or physical plane by their composition and cannot pass outside it—the life-force consciousness working in them through the Red and Orange Rays is bound within their spiritual limitations and is subject to the ordinary laws of space and time. The Etheric body is the real source of all physical vitality—the absorber of the vital fluid of life called *prana* or solar energy. The twin principles are rarely separated during earthly life, but separation does occur when certain drugs and anaesthetics are administered.

It is most important to remember that the Etheric double is an exact replica or duplicate of the visible organism, particle for particle, and the medium through which play all the electro-magnetic radiations and the vital currents on which the activity of the body depends. As we shall see, it has its own organs and centres corresponding to the same regions of the dense body.

31

The physical world consists of seven general subdivisions with a large number of combinations within its own limits and all are acted upon and influenced by the Red Cosmic Ray.

In the chemical portion of the dense body there are gases, liquids and solids ; in the invisible or Etheric portion we find the Chemical Ether, the medium for the forces of assimilation and excretion, the primary Life Ether, the medium for propagation, the Light Ether, the medium of sense perception, and the Reflectory Ether, the medium of the accumulated records of evolution.

It is not proposed to encumber the student of the inner mysteries with a mass of physiological data concerning the physical nature of man—all such information can be readily found in any up-to-date medical textbook.

The great point we would impress upon the student is that the body is a dual creature—an instrument which has to be trained, refined, harmonised with the higher elements and moulded with such a form as may best fit it to be the instrument on the physical plane for the highest purposes of man.

The student of Colour aims at linking up his physical organism with the great Cosmic Life-force which is the infinite and inexhaustible source of Health, Vitality and Energy.

In seeking to train, mould and purify the physical body, the Colour student realises that there is a set of activities that are for the most part outside the control of the Will as well as those which are under such control.

The key to the physical body is the Nervous System, which is divided into two parts. One carries on all the activities of the body for maintaining its ordinary life, by which the lungs contract, by which the heart pulsates, by which the movements of the digestive system are directed.

This is called the Involuntary Nervous System. In the first epochs of evolution this system was under the control of the animal, but it gradually began to function automatically, directed by the sub-conscious mind. The ordinary healthy person does not notice its activities ; he becomes aware of breathing when the action is oppressed or checked, he feels his heart beating when the action is defective, but when all is in order the functions go on unnoticed.

It is, however, by no means impossible to bring these sub-conscious processes under the control of the will. The practice of such systems as Yoga develops this power to an extraordinary degree, but it is not recommended for Western occultists. The Hatha Yogi is able to control his breathing to an amazing extent, and also the action of the heart, quickening or retarding the circulation at will. These exercises are intended to stimulate certain psychic faculties, and are also used to induce a condition of trance and setting free the astral body.

The complete science of Yoga is not advised or encouraged, but a much modified practice of breath-control is highly beneficial to the physical, mental and spiritual development. The system of Colour Breathing taught in this book is safe for all to practise.

The other nervous system to be considered is the great voluntary nervous system. This aspect of our physical life enables us to feel, move and think on the physical plane.

This system is centred on the cerebral-spinal axis—the brain and spinal cord—whence go to every part of the body filaments of nervous matter, the sensory and motor nerves—" the nerves of feeling " running from the outer periphery to the axis and the " nerves of movement " running from the axis to the periphery.

These nerve-lines are very complicated but are all based on the brain and the Solar Plexus, the highly important centre in the stomach, sometimes termed the second brain.

This is the system by means of which man expresses his will and his consciousness.

In the physical aspect, man can do nothing except through the brain and nervous system—if these are defective in any way then the orderly and coherent expression of the physical powers is dislocated. The materialised school of thought maintain that thought and brain-activity are inseparable processes. From the purely physical aspect this may be true, but man is the recipient of other forces than the merely physical. Account must be taken of the vast astral region which surrounds the physical world. It is well known that in certain conditions as, e.g., disease, the presence of drugs, or injury, the brain is dulled and its normal functioning hindered, with the result that the thought of the individual so affected becomes incoherent. Other diseased conditions of the physical brain affect thought also.

Aphasia is known to destroy a part of the tissue of the brain near the ear and causes a loss of word-memory and the power of expression. Although unable to articulate words he is conscious inwardly of thought-currents—he is able to think but unable to speak.

It is the *existence of thought* apart from a defective brain-centre that causes the materialistic argument to break down.

When a man is set free from the physical body with its faults and imperfections, he is able to manifest his powers unhindered.

The point we wish to impress on the student is that man is restricted in the expression of his spirit on the physical plane owing to the limitations of the physical organism, and secondly that this organism is controlled by physical laws and circumstances—if these are able to injure it they can also improve it. This is of vital importance to us in our occult development.

Every portion of our physical body is built up on cells which are defined as a unit or aggregate of matter with a surrounding wall and contents, and modified according to their functions. These cellular organisms in their turn are formed of molecules and these again of atoms, each atom being the ultimate indivisible particle of a chemical element. By combining together they form the basic material of the physical body—the gases, liquids and solids.

Each atom and cell is a living thing with its own conscious life and each group or aggregation of such atoms and cells into a more complex being is again a living entity. They form organic bodies which appear on this earth plane as the vehicles of a higher consciousness and manifest at a higher rate of vibration than anything which they know in their separated lives.

The particles existing in a body are in a continual state of flux, forming positive and negative combinations of all kinds.

Even a drop of blood is a marvellous world in miniature. It consists of numbers of living bodies, the red and white corpuscles, the white resembling very closely the ordinary amoebae (species of cells that multiply by fission). Our blood-stream swarms with protective and destructive entities, the microbes of disease and the microbes of health which attack and devour dangerous germs and impure matter.

These living cells and tiny organisms which compose our physical bodies are susceptible to changes in vibration

—they are susceptible to the forces operating from both outside and within. They are influenced especially by radiations from our own minds and also from others, from the atmosphere and the ether, from the invisible planes around us.

The Cosmic Rays and the forces of Colour which play upon our physical bodies affect the condition of the physical and etheric cells and atoms—some groups of cells are more influenced by certain Colour rays which affinitise with them, than by others.

Each of the seven Great Colour Manifestations affect certain centres of the physical body—hence the importance of the right colour environment.

CHAPTER 5

THE ETHERIC BODY

WE saw in the previous Chapter that the physical world is composed of substances vibrating within certain fixed limits to which we gave the name " matter."

We know that matter which appears so solid is really *not* solid at all. A piece of wood or a piece of glass are made up of an immense number of electrons in vibration, revolving round a central point known as a proton. Matter consists of atoms and these atoms are in turn composed of electrons and protons which are held together by electro-magnetic forces. Thus matter is built up of minute electric charges, positive and negative, not moving at random, but freely and orderly, connected together by the invisible universal elements called the ether.

The ether is an omnipresent cosmic substance filling all space and is the vehicle or medium by which all physical-etheric forces contact the earth and ourselves.

The vibrations of the ether are many and varied. One form of etheric undulation or wave-motion gives us the phenomenon we call *light*—other forms give us heat, colour, electricity, ectoplasm, etc.

This marvellous substance is perpetually conveying across space the cosmic energy which enables us to live and think.

The Ether is never at rest, it is ever in movement—it cannot be seen or felt by the physical senses, yet if it were non-existent one would be blind and cold as there would be no medium to carry the waves of light and sound, warmth and colour. Matter itself is basically etheric.

The electrons in the atoms are particles of negative electricity and the protons are considered by science as electric in their motive. Both are etheric and matter is thus only ether in a particular state of vibration.

The ether is the great connecting link between the physical senses and the higher cosmic forces. It is obvious that our physical senses only respond to a very limited range of vibrations, that outside these there is a universe full of life and thought which responds to a higher range of vibrations, unreal to us but more real to it than physical matter. Our ordinary senses—our range of sight, touch, perception, smell, hearing—are limited to the last degree. This fact is clearly illustrated by the scientific instrument known as the spectroscope which analyses light into its seven component parts. Our physical eyes perceive only an infinitesimal part of the vibrations of colour—the visible vibrations as compared with the invisible are much less than is an inch compared to a mile. It is evident that there is a vast region of force and activity beyond our normal sense perceptions. Until we realise that our ordinary senses respond to a very limited range of vibrations and that outside there is a vast universe of life and activity, we cannot hope to unfold and develop our inner perception.

The etheric forces influence physical life in a variety of ways. They are creative and formative, ensouling matter with life, vitality, form and power—the ether is the transmitter of the essential life-forces. Furthermore, this cosmic organising force is susceptible to control by Mind and Will—mind controls life and life controls matter.

Just as the physical world is surrounded and influenced by the ether, so also is man. The etheric forces are gathered and concentrated in man and form what is called the Etheric Body or double, which surrounds and interpenetrates the physical body and is an exact copy or duplicate of it, organ for organ and cell for cell.

The Etheric, or vital body, as it is also called, extends beyond the periphery of the dense body as the etheric region extends beyond the dense part of the planet.

The distance of this extension of the etheric body is about an inch and a half, and it is visible to clairvoyants as a luminous outline of a pale golden colour.

The etheric body plays a very important part in our life, health and the development of occult powers.

The vital force from the sun which surrounds us as subtle radiations is absorbed by the etheric body through the splenic centre or chakram whence it becomes transformed into a pale rose-coloured vibration and flows through the nervous system all over the body.

In health the etheric body specialises a vast amount of vital force which often, vitalising the physical body, radiates in straight lines in every direction ; during ill-health the etheric body shrinks and is unable to absorb the same amount of solar force to supply the etheric nourishment required by the physical body. In consequence, the radiations of vital force passing outwards appear drooping and bent, showing the lack of vitality. Instead of the radiant golden colour, dark grey patches and twisted spots are seen round the affected organs.

In health the etheric radiations expel inimical germs and microbes, but in ill-health these emanations are not powerful enough to be effective.

In all cases of ill-health, the natural treatment is to build up the exhausted forces in the etheric body by applying colour-vibrations to the appropriate centres. Colour is the great cosmic healing force which works directly on the etheric cells, replenishing and revitalising them.

The etheric body consists of four separate essences or ethers.

The first or lowest ether is the *Chemical Ether*—positive and negative. It is the conductor of the forces which cause assimilation and excretion. The second is the *Life Ether* and is the avenue for the forces which concern the perpetuation of the species—the forces of propagation. The forces working along the positive pole are those which work in the female during gestation, supplying the power of bringing forth a new being. The negative Life Ether enables the male to secrete semen. The third is the *Light Ether*. The positive forces of this ether generate the blood heat, individualising it in man and animal. The negative forces operate through the physical senses such as sight, hearing, feeling, etc. The Red Ray controls this ether.

In the vegetable kingdom, instead of blood the Light-ether generates the green life-substance, chlorophyl. The Light-Ether is of great importance in the manifestation of Colour in all the kingdoms of nature.

The *fourth ether* is called the Reflecting Ether—it is through the medium of this ether that thought makes an impression on the human brain. Every thought has an " etheric double "—in other words everything that has ever happened is imprinted permanently on the Reflecting Ether and because of this the psychometrist or clairvoyant is able to see or read the etheric records surrounding us.

The Reflecting Ether must not be confused with the Spiritual Akasa. In the lower reflecting ether no spiritual clairvoyant cares to read, as the records and impressions are earthy and vague, compared to those found in the higher realm. The novice in occult development in the early stages of his training often contacts this lower ether, but he has to be duly warned by his teacher concerning its inadequacy and shortcomings.

The Reflecting Ether is only the copy or reflection of what the Akasa is in the spiritual realms.

The Etheric Body being the counterpart of the physical is more often seen by developing clairvoyants than any of man's other vehicles. It is an exact copy of our outer body in every way, only it is composed of a much finer material in a higher rate of vibration. It acts as the builder and restorer of the outer body. Its etheric organs, corresponding in every way to the physical, regulate and control the functions of physical life. During life it never separates from the physical body, except in such unusual conditions as trance, catalepsy, hypnosis, etc.

The Etheric Body plays an important part in the phenomena of sleep. Sleep is caused by the cutting off temporarily of the vital ethers passing through the Etheric Body. It is as though the currents of air in a room, or of electricity through a wire, were suddenly suspended; vitality closes down. Sleep, however, is not a merely torpid state of inactivity. The higher principles of man withdraw from the physical shell into the astral and even higher realms where the work of restraining the rhythm and harmony of the Ego and its principles (the kind and astral body) is carefully attended to. They transmit the healing forces into the Etheric Body which is then able to revitalise the physical being. Beside the activities connected with the renewal of vital energy, the Ego and its principles are sometimes impressed in various ways during the sleep-state and can receive higher knowledge and guidance from the spiritual spheres.

Some dreams, but not all, are the faint and imperfect

reflections or memories of activities, whilst out of the body it should also be realised that dreaming is a power of the soul which can be developed and which can also be manipulated by spiritual beings who mould our dream-substance into symbols and impressions for our guidance and progress.

Chapter 6

COSMIC COLOUR

LIGHT and Colour, said the philosopher Bacon, demand investigation before form, for *Colour is Life*.

The splendid symphony of colour which we see manifested on all sides of the universe is the visible expression of Divine Mind. It is the cosmic manifestation of the One Life Principle in the form of Light-waves. Pythagoras declared that there is " One Universal Soul permeating all things, which in substance resembles Light."

In our universe all light is an emanation from the central sun : Colour is a mode of differentiation of this primal light according to different rates of vibration. The visible universe, as a whole, as well as each separate or organic part, manifests on the physical plane through the cosmic forces of Light, Form and Vibration.

In the Cosmos there are light-rays of a much higher order and power than the colours, or reflections, with which we are familiar. Colour expresses the very Soul of the Universe. According to Paracelsus and other great masters of the secret wisdom, when a universal life-cycle begins, it first appears as a rapidly-vibrating mass of scintillating colours—an infinite spiral of colours. Within the spiral globe resides the mighty cosmic power of transmuting spiritual energy into spiritual substance and vice versa. The great ocean of light is radiated from the central sun, the storehouse of all energies and potencies and the source of all light warmth and motion on this planet. From this fact we can appreciate the tremendous energy stored up in light and radiation.

43

In studying Colour we are studying a force of immeasureable and infinite power. The Ancient Egyptians were conscious of the power and influence of colour, and in their great temples certain parts of the buildings were set aside as Colour Halls, where the effects of colour vibrations were minutely studied and applied. The Egyptian priests, the inheritors and keepers of the esoteric wisdom of a vanished epoch, left manuscripts showing their system of Colour Science which even to-day strike us as a very excellent one. They applied the law of correspondence between the sevenfold nature of man and the sevenfold division of the solar system. Thus, the Temple Masters taught, thousands of years ago, that the primary colours Red, Yellow and Blue correspond to the body, soul (mind) and spirit of man.

This is a good classification of colours and has never been discarded, although it has been enlarged upon. Although expressed in different ways and sometimes under a variety of symbols, the occultists of the past had broadly the same basis of Colour Science as we use to-day. The Science of Colour rests on the laws of light as manifested in the Seven Major Rays. The Colour Rays are intrinsically related to the seven planes of manifestation and also to the seven major glandular centres in the human body, called the *chakras*, a Hindu term meaning " wheels of light." (See Chapter 8.)

Just as there is an esoteric (inner) and exoteric (outer) meaning to all cosmic phenomena, so there is an esoteric meaning to the outward and visible rays of light comprising the spectrum. Ordinarily speaking, the sun radiates white light-waves capable of being resolved into seven main constituent parts of different wave-lengths.

From the esoteric aspect, the White Light (Spiritual Sun) enters the consciousness of the soul through the

Aura and is diffused into its seven component colours each one infusing the appropriate soul-centre with power and vitality.

Each Major Colour has seven intrinsic elements, viz. :

1. A physical or material element.
2. A vitality-giving power (life-force).
3. A psychological element.
4. An harmonising, unifying element.
5. A specific healing element.
6. An element of inspiration and intuition.
7. A spiritual or higher-consciousness element.

In the ordinary sense, the Seven Major Rays are known as :

1. Red
2. Orange
3. Yellow   These colours should be visualised
4. Green   mentally daily until they can be sensed
5. Blue   in the mind.
6. Indigo
7. Violet

These names of the colours like the numerals alongside them are in reality the symbols or veils of hidden powers and forces of great significance.

The tabulation of colours given above concerns only the octave of visible light. At each end of the spectrum there exist several octaves of higher radiations and X-radiations, admitted by physical science, and beyond them are the Cosmic Rays.

The Seven Major Rays signify a great deal more than vibratory waves of light. Cosmically speaking, the spectrum is an epitome of the evolution of our Universe.

Each of the seven rays stands for one of the great evolutionary epochs. In reality, the Rays are forces of infinite power and purpose emanating from the Supreme Source, the great White Light, and guided and directed by all-powerful intelligences. The Rays illumine and sustain the human soul. The word " soul " is derived from Sol (sun) and is the light-centre within our being. In the Seven Spirits of the Rays are centred all the potentialities of Absolute Being.

The whole planet—the oceans, the earth, everything we see manifested as mineral, plant, animal and human forms —is dependent upon Light and its amazing properties and radiations for its very existence. Not only the physical world—our material earth plane—but the higher worlds constituting our universe, the etheric, astral, mental and spiritual planes, depend upon the same source of Light and each have their own rate of vibration.

Referring again to the Seven Major Rays, the occultist sees in them an ascending scale in the progress of evolution. The first three periods corresponding to the Red, Orange, and Yellow Rays have already been passed through. We are now in the fourth or Green Ray epoch midway between the lower periods of struggle and bitter experience and the higher periods of soul-growth and spiritual faculties.

The Cosmic Wisdom teaches that we have now reached the nadir of materiality—the outlook of the future is an upward advance into the higher vibration of the Blue Ray, and then an advance slowly towards the finer and more ethereal conditions of the Indigo and Violet Rays.

We should always be mindful of the fact that we are surrounded at all times by Cosmic Colour. The vast ocean of consciousness in which we live is vibrating with life and colour and is capable of receiving and transmitting thought. The great cosmic currents or Rays of Force are the real source of our powers, abilities, talents and so-called natural gifts. In one aspect, the Cosmic Rays cause material success and fulfilment in life, in another they impart artistic, musical or literary ability, in another they furnish the power for performing cures and restoring health. All healing systems and processes, whatever their name may be, work under the same law and through the same Force.

The true Cosmic Rays are spiritual forces emanating from the Divine White Light. The Rays are perpetually vibrating not only on the surface of the earth, but also above and through it, encircling the globe in streams of endless, inexhaustible energy. As in the macrocosm so also in microcosm—the same rays and forces surround and permeate every human being, flowing down the negative left side of the body and up the positive right side, for man is a miniature world.

This is not mere fancy or day-dreaming. Dr. Edwin Babbitt, one of the chief Colour-scientists of modern times, developed the power of cosmic colour-perception. In his book, *Principles of Light and Colour*, he relates his experiences in the following words : " I commenced cultivating in a dark room and with closed eyes my interior vision, and in a few months was able to see those glories of Light and Colour which no tongue can describe or intelligence conceive of—unless they have been seen. After seeing these, when I opened my eyes upon the sky and earth around me they seemed colourless, dim and feeble.

" Sometimes fountains of light would flow out from me and become lost to view in the distance. More generally, flashing streams of light would move to and fro in a straight line, though sometimes fluidic emanations would sweep around in curves of a parabola as in a fountain. What was more marvellous than anything else was the infinite millions of radiations, emanations and luminous currents which at all times would seem streaming FROM and INTO and THROUGH all things and filling all the surrounding space with coruscations and lighting activities. I believe that if the amazing streams of forces which sweep in all directions could suddenly be revealed to people many untutored souls would go wild with fright."

Colour is a cosmic power and therefore a vital, stupendous force. It works through and in us, in every nerve, cell gland and muscle : it shines in our Auras and radiates upon us from the atmosphere. In our higher bodies, Colour is an active power, exerting a tremendous influence on the consciousness, the soul and the spirit.

The value of a force such as Colour is that in essence it is spiritual. Theoretically speaking, there is no need for any material equipment or appliances, although they are a useful aid in augmenting colour-treatments.

SUMMARY

(To form the basis of Affirmations)

1. Colour is a Vital Force. It is a manifestation of Divine Mind. It is the original cosmic vibration.
2. Colour oppresses the Soul of the Universe. It radiates from the Central Sun like a great Ocean of Light.
3. The Seven Major Rays fill space and permeate my Soul and Being. They correspond to the Seven Major Glandular Centres in my body.
4. In the Spirit of the Rays exist all the potentialities of Cosmic Consciousness.

Chapter 7

THE BASIS OF TREATMENT BY COLOUR

THE source of all terrestrial life—the Sun—contains within it practically everything of which the earth is composed. The colours revealed in the spectroscope are indicative of various metals and gases given off in the forms of ethers which vary in intensity and quality, some of these forces being termed heat or thermal, and others cold or electric. The trinity of colours Red, Yellow and Blue have a definite correspondence with the three basic elements, hydrogen, carbon, and oxygen, which form so large a proportion of life on our globe.

The use of coloured glass prevents certain rays passing through and when these are shut off certain definite results are produced. The effect of colour on vegetable life, for instance, shows some very interesting results. In experiments with lettuce it has been ascertained that the plant grows four times as quickly under red glass as compared to ordinary sunlight. Under green glass the result was less striking, yet the lettuce was taller than that grown in sunlight : under blue light the results were quite negligible. If the vegetable kingdom responds to the radiation contained in coloured glass, why not the animal ? The tests and experiments that have been carried out have adequately justified the inference.

Scientists and savants of the calibre of Camille Flammarion, Dr. Edwin Babbitt, Dr. Ponza, Dr. Pancoast, Dr. Kilner, Dr. Barraduc and numerous others have established very amply the case for colour radiation in health and disease.

DIAGNOSIS

The Colour Healer employs both physical and super-physical methods of diagnosis. Of the two the super-physical aspect is the more important as it is concerned with *causes*, whereas the physical method merely concerns the observation of symptoms.

The superphysical method is so-called because it deals with the conditions which lie over and behind the physical —in other words, it seeks to penetrate to the root of the trouble. The constitution of man is very complex owing to the sevenfold planes or levels of consciousness, each plane requiring a separate body or vehicle. The sum-total of man's inner being is expressed or outpictured in the Aura, the radiation surrounding and interpenetrating every individual. This colour-atmosphere is the key to the condition prevailing in the physical, etheric, astral, mental and spiritual life-aspects of the man. It reflects the condition of health, the superfluities or deficiencies, and the localisation of disease.

Disease manifests in the Aura in certain defined ways such as dark patches or spots over the organs affected, greyness, paleness, bent or deflected rays. In health the lines of vital force radiate in straight lines and project emanations of vitality and vigour. Auric diagnosis pre-supposes the power of clairvoyance or some degree of sensing-power in the healer, such as intuition. Advanced healers know intuitively the exact level of consciousness wherein the disease originates. The personal presence of the patient is not essential as his condition can be sensed from any object he has held or from a photograph.

In place of clairvoyance or intuition the device origi-nated by Dr. Kilner is a useful substitute. Dr. Kilner realised that if the auric radiations were really perceptible to specially sensitive sight they belonged to the ultra-violet range of light. This type of light is normally invisible to sight, being of a wave-length that is too short or of a vibratory rate that is too high for ordinary vision. He therefore constructed a screen to exclude certain light-rays and to render the ultra-violet visible. Concisely speaking, it consisted of a glass-screen containing an alcoholic solution of decyanin, a coal-tar dye.

The subject under observation is placed against a dark background in a dimly-lighted room. The observer prepares his auric sight by gazing through the screen for a few moments at a fairly bright light, preferably a north sky on a sunny day, or in lieu of that, at a 100-watt electric bulb : then before the light coming through the dye-solution wears off he concentrates intently on the subject.

The Kilner Screen is valuable for observing the etheric and astral Auras, but does not appear to extend to the mental and higher Auras.

A further method of diagnosis is to pass the fingers of the right (positive) hand over the patient's body, gently and lightly, until the healer senses a vibration or an oscillation of the finger-tips indicating the position of the disease. In the system of Radiesthesia a light pendulum is used.

DIAGNOSIS BY PHYSICAL METHODS

Observation of the physical symptoms of a patient is the main feature in the second type of diagnosis. The healer should bear in mind that the two basic colours used in Chromopathy are Red and Blue—the thermal and the cooling. These two colours form the basic vibrations in every human being and the aim of the healer is to discern which of the two vibrations is lacking.

The main physical signs of a lack of the Red Ray are

seen when a man is deficient in energy, rich blood, appetite or if he suffers from constipation, etc. The secondary indications are sleepiness and general inactive disposition. When the Blue Ray is absent there are signs of over-activity, fussiness, irritability, feverishness, etc.

System of Treatment

The basis of treatment, whether physical or super-physical, is the restoring and re-charging of the body-cells with the correct colour vibration through the glandular centres or chakras. The remedial rays may be radiated (1) from a lamp or reflector to be absorbed by the etheric body ; (2) projected into the mental Aura so as to cause a change of consciousness and thought ; (3) inhaled from the atmosphere by correct breathing ; (4) absorbed into the body from the elements contained in certain foods and light-charged liquids.

Broadly speaking there are two main factors producing disease, viz.: physical and non-physical. Disease is said to be of physical origin when it results from the wrong living, working or climatic conditions, the spread of infection, etc. Disease which results from the wrong mental, emotional and spiritual outlook and consciousness is of non-physical origin.

In general terms disease may be defined as a *condition of discord* in the cells of the bodies which the Life-force uses. It is disharmony in matter, a disintegration pre-venting the free flow of the Cosmic Life Rays and shutting off the Divine White Light. It is a condition of disturbance of equilibrium and is unstable, negative and impermanent. Disease has no place in Colour-harmonies and cannot attach itself to Health.

Radiant Colour is a polarised, vital force. In the abso-lute aspect, Light and Colour are controlled by groups of intelligent entities who share in the work of helping humanity. The seven great Cosmic Rays are not the result of mere fortuitous splitting up of light, but are the active agents for the good of mankind, designed and emanated by high creative intelligence.

If Health remains potential in the atoms of the body, if it is inactive or frustrated, then disease—disharmony, lack of equilibrium—may become dominant in the system. But if the Colour Rays can fill the diminished centres and open a channel through the etheric and other bodies which will make an inlet for the regenerating White Light so as to change and raise the unstable vibrations and establish its own cosmic equilibrium, then disease is no longer active.

Health is the true condition of man's spiritual being— an aspect of the all-pervading Life Itself. It is a normal inherent power and may be said to be a Law of the great Creator for all things in manifestation, for every conscious entity. In its source Health is spiritual and absolute and cannot separate from its own nature nor identify itself with that which is not of the same rate of vibration as itself.

The science of colour teaches us that Colours, like other forces and energies in Nature, may be either positive or negative in its effect, either beneficial or harmful, according to the circumstances. It is, therefore, of the utmost importance that we should cultivate the right colour vibrations in our personal lives and surroundings. A great deal of the discord and antagonism between members of families and groups of people closely associated together arises from cross-vibrations due to inharmonious colour combinations within the personal Aura and environment.

CHAPTER 8

THE CHAKRAS

IN this Chapter we will consider the seven Chakras and their relation to the colour principles in man.

We have seen that Solar Energy is the source of all forms of energy in our Universe. Scientists have discerned that in sunlight there exist certain particles which contain a special vital and stimulatory force. These particles are termed *vitality globules*. Eastern occultists have long known these globules of life under the generic name of *prana*, which literally means breath, or life.

In the human body *prana* is specialised by each individual when it is drawn into the body from the atmosphere through the chakras and distributed over the whole system. The vital energy in prana is present in every cell and molecule of the body.

The chakras are bell-shaped vortices appearing in the etheric body (the vital counterpart of the physical). These vortices have a characteristic colour and intersect the spinal cord at certain definite points.

There are seven major chakras in the human body and some subsidiary ones. Thus the Violet Chakram is situated at the top of the head in the region of the pituitary gland. The Indigo Chakram is behind the mid-forehead controlling the pineal body. The Blue Chakram lies within the throat and is based on the thyroid gland. The Green Chakram is situated at the cardiac plexus—the heart. The Yellow Chakram, the golden centre, lies in the Solar plexus, influencing the adrenal glands, the pancreas and

54

the liver. The Orange Chakram is centred in the spleen, and the Red Chakram, the coccygeal centre, at the base of the spine.

It should be noted that the Red and Orange Chakras, which have to do with the physical and etheric aspects in man, are very closely related and are sometimes classed together as a single unit. The size and configuration of the chakras depends on the type of individual and the genesial stage of development. The more evolved his astial, mental and spiritual aspects are the clearer and more definite the chakras become and the more perfect their colours. Concisely speaking, they are the etheric organs working through thought and feeling directly upon the physical body.

The chakras are specialised channels of Colour force. Each chakram absorbs a special current of vital energy through its particular Colour ray from the physical environment and from higher levels of consciousness. The Orange Chakram, for example, draws in the prana of the physical atmosphere, i.e., the sunlight with its life-giving vitality globules.

The vital energy of the Orange Ray is absorbed and distributed to all parts of the body.

Whilst this higher prana-energy is not inhaled through the lungs the activity of the Orange Chakram is directly associated with breathing. Its activity is determined by the breathing rhythm which increases the absorption of vitality globules.

Deep rhythmic breathing is of great value—it enables us to draw in a much greater supply of physical prana than the shallow, unmeasured form of breathing.

The most beneficial form is Colour Breathing. It will be found most vitalising and uplifting and a general tonic for tired minds and nerves.

In Colour Breathing one mentally visualises the life-giving radiations of Colour pouring in from the atmosphere surrounding us.

The simplest way is to sit upright on a chair before an open window. Slowly relax the body by bending forward, with the arms limp, and exhale all the air from your lungs. Then breathe in slowly, as you resume an upright position, focusing your mind on the Indigo Chakram (the pineal body within the forehead). The breath must be held whilst you count from one to twelve calmly and unhurriedly. You will soon find that the counting becomes automatic whilst your conscious mind dwells on the thought of new power, life and harmony flooding your entire being. Later on as you make progress, it is greatly beneficial to breathe deeply to a universal affirmation, visualising the colour you desire to manifest in your Aura. The great advantage of this exercise is that it replenishes your whole being with new life and also develops the power of seeing the Aura.

Occult science teaches that the supply of prana is greater in direct light—perfectly natural or artificial sunlight—but deep rhythmic Breathing anywhere increases the flow of vitality.

Thirty seconds of deep breathing can change the appearance of the health Aura for the time being, transforming it from grey to deep blue, strengthening the emanations and restoring them from a bent droopy condition to straight rays of power and health.

The other chakras influence the appropriate centres on different planes. Each one acts as a channel for a particular influence from one or other of the psychological centres.

Thus the Orange Chakram, in the splenic centre, influences the emotional or astral nature of man, as also does the Yellow Chakram in a greater or lesser degree.

It should be remembered that no two individuals are ever exactly alike. The psychological influences vary exceedingly and the activity of the chakras are not strictly localised but are interpenetrative.

Strictly speaking, the Yellow Chakram (Solar Plexus) is the centre of the lower mind (objective, material) and is also complicated by emotional influences.

Golden Yellow is the colour of intellect in its various phases and aspect.

The Green Chakram (heart) registers impulses of the higher mind (subjective, abstract) and also higher emotions, such as compassion and sympathy.

The Blue Chakram (throat) is the gateway to the spiritual aspect of man. It is the centre of the religious instinct, the devotional and mystical nature. When working in harmony with the Yellow and Red Chakras, there is peace and balance in body and mind. It is the home of the casual body—the root cause of your present condition of life.

The two higher chakras are super-rational and transcendental—their activity is generally found only in initiates or highly developed souls. The Indigo Chakram presides over the higher phenomena of the soul—sensitivity, spiritual perception and intuition true occult forces, clairvoyance, power of vision, healing, etc.

Its root-centre is the pineal gland.

The Violet Chakram at the crown of the head is the sanctuary of the Spirit, the gateway to the highest spiritual influences in man. Its material counterpart is the pituitary body.

CHAPTER 9

METHODS OF TREATMENT

COLOUR THERAPY. LAMP RADIATION

ONE of the best ways of using Colour for the treatment of specified ills or for the restoration of health is by employing some simple apparatus, such as an electric Colour Lamp or some coloured glass. The latter is somewhat difficult to obtain now but simple colour lamps are procurable. They are made to focus the seven rays as required.

Whatever type of light projector is used the same principles apply. There are two main kinds of Ray treatment, viz. : general diffusion and local concentration. In general diffusion the light-rays are focused on the body, especially the back, the region of the spine and nervous system. General diffusion is excellent for re-charging the tired nerve cells with new life. The patient either sits or lies down in a relaxed position, stripped to the waist, and is wholly immersed in the light for thirty minutes. Colour treatment by lamps should not exceed this period. An auxiliary to general diffusion is Radiant Magnetism.

In local concentration the light is focused on the affected area only. The great value of colour-therapy lies in the penetrative power of light. Light and Colour have a direct action on the protoplasm of the body—the speed and power of the chemical reactions depend upon the biological state of the organism.

Radiation is still a subject that is little understood and the penetrating properties of certain cosmic rays are even more marvellous than those of light. The Cosmic Rays rain upon the earth in continuous showers from outer space and contain charged-particles of enormous energy. Their penetrating power is so great that the rays have been detected in mines 3,000 ft. under the earth.

Exactly how light penetrates or influences the body is not easy to comprehend. One view is that a permeation of the cells takes place as in ordinary osmosis. The most favoured view, however, is that light and colour influence the body by arousing sympathetic vibrations within the organism. In other words light and colour work according to the Law of Attraction.

In studying the nature of light it is important to remember that all radiations emitted from a luminous body travel through space in perfect rhythmic vibrations in the form of waves. The point or distance from crest to crest is called the wave-length and their " best " or rate of vibration is known as their frequency. Colours have varying wave-lengths. For instance, Violet consists of very short waves, while Red has much longer ones. These facts are important in treating disease. The deep, slow, warming vibration of Red light stimulates and invigorates the system, while the shorter and higher Violet and Blue waves calm and pacify.

As a wave of light is projected through space it creates a certain rhythm—an harmonious vibration of etheric matter. When light and colour strike a surface the homogeneous particles are thrown into sympathetic vibration with the incoming current : as a result the organism is vitalised and recharged. If, however, the particles within the body are non-conductive or of an opposite rate of vibration, or if the power of the incoming current is too strong, then an abnormal reaction will occur which may produce serious harm or damage. It is very important for the healer to know the nature of the light or colour he uses—its quality, quantity or intensity.

The essence of Colour-healing consists in causing certain molecular reactions in the organism or vital centres through the medium of the rays. Light, it should be remembered, is not a force or energy outside us—light enters into the centre of every cell, nerve and tissue of our bodies. Nature has given us this wonderful form of energy which is the basis of life, to maintain our minds and bodies alike in perfect health.

COLOUR BREATHING

Just as the invisible radiations of the sun and the Cosmic Rays surround us on all sides, so also the very air we breathe is permeated with the forces of light and colour. This vital energy, or *prana*, as the Hindus call it, is the living force that imparts and sustains life. We extract it from the food we eat, from the water we drink and most of all from the air we breathe. When we absorb large quantities of prana we enjoy good health and vitality.

What we call " fresh air " consists of much more than just oxygen and other chemical ingredients. It contains radiations from the sun, from the far-off stars and planets as well as from the earth. Air is the outer vehicle of prana and other forces. The Colour Healer therefore practises deep rhythmic breathing with visualisation of the rays absorbing them into his body and inner principles. He also teaches his patients to practice deep breathing, and to make simple mental affirmations expressive of the Ray being drawn upon.

The Colour Healer is always a deep breather. He is always conscious of the Universal Life-Spirit that is about him to strengthen him and with each deep inbreathing he draws into himself a portion of this power. He does this consciously feeling the grandeur of being in harmony with the Infinite. When he eats it is with the feeling that he is taking sustenance into his body which is adding to his reserve force. When he sleeps it is with the knowledge that he entrusts himself to the beneficent action of Divine Energy in rebuilding the exhausted cells of the body and inspiring him for the tasks of the next day.

The following exercise will be found most useful and beneficial. Sit comfortably in a chair before an open window : close your eyes and when you have contemplated in the mind for three minutes on the desired colour, bend forward and expel all the air from your lungs and stomach, making the body as limp as possible. All the muscles must be relaxed so that each limb is perfectly limp and as far as possible forgotten. Then take one deep inbreathing beginning with the expansion of the abdomen and carrying the breath up by one continued inspiration inhalation to the ribs and chest. As you breathe in count up to eight : then hold the breath for another eight seconds and lastly exhale during eight more seconds.

The best time to practise is immediately following or preceding breakfast and supper. The exercise should not be practised last thing at night during the first month as it is definitely stimulating and the increase of vital force may take some time to get accustomed to. It is important to feel conscious during this exercise of the inflow of the rays revitalising the whole system and replenishing the finer vehicles with cosmic energy. Controlled breathing not only raises the bodily vibrations but unites us subjectively with the Universal Consciousness.

Each of the seven rays may be breathed in according to the specific need. It is well to remember that the first

three Colour Rays, i.e., Red, Orange, Yellow, are magnetic, and should be visualised as flowing up from the
earth towards the solar plexus. The last three—Blue,
Indigo, Violet—are electrical and are breathed in from the
ether downwards. The Green Ray—the balancer of the
spectrum—flows into the system horizontally.

RADIANT MAGNETISM

Many scientists who have studied the invisible forces
of the human system have come to the conclusion that the
body is similar to a magnet. Reichenbach, Dr. Kilner,
Dr. Baraduc, Dr. Babbitt and others speak of the luminous
emanations which have been seen flowing from the finger-
tips of healers and sensitives. The hands are the main
source of healing magnetism and are the channels of the
seven rays.

To quote the words of Dr. Gregory, author of *Animal
Magnetism* : " The human body is found to possess the
same influence and to produce the same effects as magnets.
I have already spoken of the light seen to issue from the
tips of the operator's fingers. The hands are oppositely
polar, and the head, eyes and mouth are also foci where
the auric influence seems to be concentrated." (Page 100,
Animal Magnetism.)

The right or positive hand is used for transmitting the
healing vibrations into the patient's body : the left or
negative hand is used to close the circuit and also to draw
off the negative conditions of the patient. The value of
the hand in healing is well expressed by Dr. Coates in
his book, *Human Magnetism* : " The human hand is used
instinctively in the alleviation of pain and in the cure of
disease. The whole process is perfectly natural whether
applied to self-healing or to the healing of others. If a
person suffers from cramp in the stomach, in the side or in

a limb, immediately the hand flies to the spot, and by rubbing, manipulation of and about the region affected, the cramp is removed. In headache and in toothache the involuntary application of the hand is a common occurrence. The operation is hereditary or instinctive so that in spite of scepticism I have known a doctor nurse his own head or jaw, seeking relief in this manner, and while it is probable that he was not in a condition to benefit himself, yet another person in a state of health and possessed of sufficient sympathy, laying hands on the affected part could give help and perhaps cure the disease."

Dr. Coates was able to put restless and sleepless patients to sleep by merely laying his hand upon their brows. "The hand soothed pain and the hand gave sleep : therefore from the hand or by the hand was conveyed to the sufferer something which was needed, something also that I was fortunately able to impart." (Page 114, *Human Magnetism*.)

The advanced healer can consciously direct the correct colour-current through his sensitive hands. As a general rule the right hand should be placed over the solar plexus, whilst the left hand is held over the chakram or glandular centre requiring healing treatment.

The solar plexus is a great nerve-centre exercising an important influence on the health. The application of the positive hand on this plexus causes the healing ray to radiate through the entire nervo-vital system from head to foot—thence it sets in the direction of the healer's left hand, seeking to complete the circuit. When the healer feels that the circuit has been completed he withdraws his left hand from the spinal centre or wherever it may be resting and allows the colour-vibration to flow into his patient from the right hand alone. This may take from one to five minutes. After a short pause he taps the centre or organ with the tip of the third finger of his left hand. This causes a flow of colour-magnetism to the point of contact and should result in a sensation similar to a mild current of electricity. The healer allows his finger to rest in one place for a few seconds and then proceeds to touch the spinal cord from end to end. This should continue for five minutes.

It is important to administer the treatment with warm hands—if cold they should be first rubbed briskly together before applying them to the patient. In all treatments the patient should close his eyes and cultivate a relaxed condition of mind and body.

THE COLOUR PASS

For receiving this treatment the patient sits comfortably in a chair, thoroughly relaxed, with eyes closed. A few words on relaxation may be given before the commencement. The healer then stands in front of the patient and concentrates on the colour he wishes to transmit. He makes a mental affirmation such as : " I will restore colour and health to this patient, or, I will relieve the patient of his pain. I will transmit such-or-such colour ray to restore his nervous system to harmony."

While so concentrating, he slowly raises both hands, with the fingers clenched, and in a wide sweep raises them above the patient's head, bringing them together and unclenching the fingers at a point just above his forehead. He next spreads his fingers out a little and very slowly brings them down past the forehead, face, chest, abdomen to the knees, taking a full thirty seconds for the movement. The healer's body follows the downward sweep of the hands. After the complete pass shake the hands to throw off the negative vibrations of the patient, then clench the fingers again and repeat the process. The treatment should be continued for five minutes.

This is an ideal way to transmit colour-vibrations when apparatus is lacking. Remember that the Red and Orange Rays increase the vitality, the Yellow Rays supply nerve power, the Green Rays soothe and energise, the Blue Rays induce calmness and spiritual inspiration, bringing the higher consciousness into activity.

The hands are the only instruments used in this general treatment for transferring colour to a patient and both hands should be employed in every case.

COLOUR-CHARGED CLOTHS

When treating patients living at a distance it is a great aid in supplementing the absent treatment to forward a piece of cloth polarised to the individual healing ray. Take a piece of coloured silk or cloth about the size of a postcard and sprinkle it with a few drops of water on both sides. Place it between the palms of your hands for two minutes, concentrating your mind upon it and willing strongly that the colour rays shall be absorbed and passed on to your patient. It should be sent wrapped in clean paper and should be worn by the patient on the part of the body requiring treatment. No one but the patient should handle the magnetised cloth.

Regarding the magnetisation of objects, Dr. Babbitt states : " In cool weather when the air is electrical I can make one, two or three strokes over tissue or other paper, and throwing it into the air within a foot of the wall, it will spring to it like a thing of life and cling there for hours, sometimes even for days. A mere stroke will make it attractive of everything around it, although it will generally repel another magnetised sheet, unless this sheet is magnetised with the same stroke as they lie together. Thousands of others can do the same thing and some better than myself." (*Principles of Light and Colour*, page 429.)

MAGNETISED WATER

Most patients derive benefit from water that has been magnetised or ray-charged. Take a glass and fill it with cold water : hold the glass in the left hand and place the right hand over it with the fingers and thumb pointing downwards over the surface of the water but not touching it. Now concentrate upon the healing colour you desire to instil into the water. Five minutes' concentration will magnetise a glass of water with colour-vibrations. The patient should take the water in doses of a wineglassful every half-hour for the first day, every hour for the second day, and a wineglassful three times a day to finish the treatment.

As an interesting experiment it is suggested that the healer sets two glasses of water before a patient, one of which has been magnetised, and allow him to distinguish between the two. Patients usually declare that the magnetised water has a slightly metallic taste.

WARM INSUFFLATION (A very ancient healing method)

The vital force contained in the breath has previously been mentioned. The mouth being a focus of human magnetism and colour radiation, the advanced healer is able to transmit healing force by breathing upon the patient. Warm insufflation is given by breathing upon a piece of flannel laid upon the affected area. The healer places his mouth close against the flannel and by breathing heavily upon it causes heat-vibrations to be felt in the part. The breathing is continued several minutes. This method is found effective in relieving many forms of nerve pains, such as headaches, neuralgia and rheumatism —in fact, any acute pain. Chronic constipation also responds to the breathing treatment. Place a piece of flannel about six inches square on the bare skin over the solar plexus. Bend over the patient and apply your left hand to the lumbar (lower) region of the spine so that the patient lies upon that hand.

Now breathe through the flannel with the mouth upon it, inhaling air through the nostrils. The magnetic radiation has an immediate effect on the peristaltic action and will overcome a habit of constipation of many years' standing.

Solarised Foods

One of the best ways of absorbing colour is the judicious use of vegetables, fruit and liquids that have been sun-charged. Fruit and vegetables are the direct result of the sun's radiation. The Colour Healer therefore studies the different groups of vegetables and fruit and classifies them according to the Rays to which they belong.

People need a constant replenishment of the particular rate of energy indicated by their Ray. Thus people who are polarised to the Orange Ray and who are thereby specially prone to suffer from nervous debility, kidney and splenic troubles, require plenty of Orange Ray vegetables and fruit, such as carrots, swedes, oranges, peaches. The juices and liquid extracts from these food-groups are also highly valuable.

The guiding principle in diet should be to eat the finer kinds of foods as much as possible in preference to coarse foods and to seek first those foods that contain most of the Cosmic Solar Energy.

HEALING BOWLS AND JARS

To those who do not scorn to learn from the past, I would like to mention a healing device practised by the Ancient Egyptians. The mysterious people of the Nile who worshipped the sun as a symbol of Deity knew also the power of the solar rays to rebuild the health. The priests used bowls in which the juices of certain fruits and vegetables were first expressed, and then set them out in the sun to become charged with the " energy of Ra."

They sometimes encrusted the healing bowls with jewels of the same colour as the fruit or vegetable being used to add a still greater potency. Nowadays the Colour Healer follows the same principle by using coloured glass jars corresponding to the fruit or the Rays required for the cure.

CHAPTER 10

USES OF THE SEVEN RAYS

THE RED RAY

RED is a heating, vitalising and stimulating vibration with a direct effect on the etheric centre governing the physical vitality. It is excellent in all blood-deficiency diseases, but should be used with care.

In every treatment with Colour the Healer first affirms and then projects mentally the universal harmony colour—Rose Red.

ANAEMIA

Persuade the patient to practise the Red Colour Breathing with mental affirmation. Colour in diet is very important in this treatment. Encourage the patient to eat as many Red Ray foods as possible (fruits and vegetables) and see that he drinks plenty of Red-rayed water between meals. Red light should be administered with the colour-lamp, the patient lying on his back under a sheet. Project the light first on the soles of the feet and then on the Red Chakram at the base of spine at a distance of about six inches. A second lamp of Orange Light should be directed upon the Orange Chakram (spleen) for twenty minutes. The Red Light treatment progresses in stages from the soles of the feet to the calves, knees, thighs, base of spine, allowing five to ten minutes at each stage.

The Red treatment should be followed by a few minutes of Green or Blue Light. The above treatment is also effective in cases of physical debility, exhaustion, depletion and bad circulation.

PARALYSIS

Usually caused by some mental or emotional shock or frustration. In its incipient stages Paralysis responds well to Colour Ray treatment. Readjustment of the mental attitude is the main preliminary factor. Yellow in some form should radiate constantly on the patient to build up mind power.

Administer Purple Light to the base chakram for ten minutes, the patient lying face downwards. Then proceed with the ray along the spine to the solar plexus, allowing five minutes for the light to concentrate. Afterwards the soles of the feet should be exposed for fifteen minutes to the Purple Light. Exposure of the legs and knees for ten minutes is also beneficial. Indigo light should also be radiated upon the solar plexus and the throat for five minutes.

Psychological treatment is an integral part of the treatment. A speedy cure is not to be expected in paralytic cases—a great deal will depend on the patient's own mind and attitude. The continued use of Radiant Magnetism and Etheric Massage is of great assistance.

CONSUMPTION

Give Red Light treatment and diet as in Anaemia with exposure of the chest and back for ten minutes. Alternate with Mental-healing and Radiant Magnetism. Encourage the hope, fortitude and cheerfulness of the patient.

THE ORANGE RAY

Orange is a warm, positive and stimulating colour, influencing primarily the vital processes of assimilation and circulation. It regulates the intake of food and is based on the spleen. The Orange vibrations are essential for health and vitality.

DEBILITY (Nervous and Mental)

General diffusion and local concentration of Orange Light on the solar plexus and the base of the brain for ten to fifteen minutes, followed by five minutes' exposure to Green Light. Encourage the patient to practise Orange Ray Breathing regularly with mental affirmations of positive and constructive qualities—Vitality, Energy, Power, Endurance, etc. Employ Radiant Magnetism.

ASTHMA

Observation and experience show that incorrect breathing is one of the underlying causes of this distressing complaint. It is therefore important to instruct the patient in deep Colour Breathing—the muscles of the stomach must be freely used. The mental attitude is very important in effecting a cure, as asthmatic subjects are usually prone to negative thinking—despondency, fear, pessimism, etc. Deep rhythmic breathing is an excellent fear-dispeller. Administer Orange Light on the chest and throat ten minutes at a time.

The patient should take half a wineglassful of orange-rayed water every fifteen minutes for one hour. Whenever possible the water should be set in the sun first for ten minutes. The " amber " fruit and vegetable group should be freely partaken of, especially oranges. When the final stage of the disease appears to be passing an exposure of the throat for fifteen minutes to Blue Light will be found beneficial. Radiant Magnetism may be applied if the condition seems to warrant it and the spine should be tapped with the fingers of the left hand from top to bottom : right hand on the solar plexus.

BRONCHITIS

The Orange Ray is very efficacious but rapid recovery is not to be expected in chronic cases. The Orange Light should be focused on the stomach and abdomen regularly.

Orange juice and lemon water are very helpful.

Regular and systematic Colour Breathing must be followed.

Encourage optimism, cheerfulness, perseverance.

PHLEGM

When this occurs in excess wet cough results. The chest should be exposed to Orange Light and orange-rayed water should be taken internally. Two doses in the morning and one in the evening. Phlegm formation rapidly disappears under Orange Treatment.

EPILEPSY

An explosion of nervous energy in the form of convulsion. The result is a brooding state of fear and anxiety and a devitalisation of the nerves and vital functions. Orange-rayed water is a great help as an internal remedy. The best light to use is Blue Light on the head.

When the epilepsy has been of very long duration the brain tissue becomes seriously impaired and a cure is highly problematic. Instruct the patient in Colour Principles and Psychology.

THE YELLOW RAY

Yellow is a positive magnetic vibration with a tonic effect on the nerves. The Colour also influences the higher mind and soul : it is definitely inspiring and stimulating.

The solar plexus (centre of the Yellow Chakram) is the organising brain of the nervous system. This Ray cleanses and purifies the whole system. Its affinitive colours are Green and Blue.

DYSPEPSIA.—Irritable condition of the nervous system.

Dyspepsia may be caused by either an excess of Red in the system or an excess of Blue. People who draw too much of the Red Ray into their constitutions are usually lean and haggard, whilst an excess of Blue causes the subject to be fat and phlegmatic. The treatment consists in practising deep breathing with Yellow Ray Affirmation and the drinking of yellow-rayed water frequently during the day (dose : half a wineglassful). The solar plexus should be exposed to Yellow Light for thirty minutes twice daily. Remember that the antidote to excess of Red is the Blue vibration. Blue reduces stomach irritation and restores normal digestion.

DIABETES

The fat cells form too rapidly, causing blood-impoverishment. Yellow Light should be focused on the solar plexus centre and yellow-rayed water taken twice daily. This colour-treatment will reduce the formation of fat and will give the blood a chance. As the fat cells are checked the thirst-craving diminishes. This disease causes great depletion of the etheric forces and prolonged treatment is necessary.

FLATULENCE

Yellow-charged water sipped slowly between meals is of great benefit. When high temperature is present Blue Light and blue-rayed water should be used.

Constipation

The stimulating and penetrating radiation of Yellow Light is highly beneficial in its action on the bowels. Yellow Ray Breathing should also be practised and small doses of Yellow-rayed water should be taken frequently between meals. Focus the light on the stomach region—twenty minutes morning and evening.

The Green Ray

The Green Ray is a vibration of harmony and balance—hence it is of fundamental importance to the nervous system. Nature radiates this colour perpetually and it appears midway in the solar spectrum as the point of colour-balance. Soothing and sympathetic, it does not excite, inflame or irritate. The Green Chakram is situated at the heart where the Ray exercises a strong influence on the control of the blood supply and distribution. Green is the restorer of tired nerves and the giver of new energy. It is Nature's master tonic.

Heart Complaints and Blood Pressure

Mental Healing with positive thought-rays attuned to the Green Ray is efficacious. Most heart diseases have their root-cause in the emotional body. Instruct the patient in the Rose-red Breathing Affirmation concurrently with the Green Ray. Emerald Green should be visualised and meditated upon. Focus Green Light on the heart centre. In the cases of low blood-pressure the Green Radiation should be dark and the exposure should last for thirty minutes per treatment. Green-rayed water should be taken between meals. In high blood-pressure a pale green light is used. Plenty of green vegetables should be included in the diet.

HEADACHES (Neuralgic)

Relax completely on a couch in a soothing Green Light. The whole nervous system responds readily to the Green Ray. Successful cure cannot be long delayed.

THE BLUE RAY

Dr. Edwin Babbitt in his treatise on Light and Colour says : " The Blue Ray is one of the greatest antiseptics in the world." Blue is a cold vibration with astringent and sleep inducing properties. It is an " electric ray." Both in its positive and negative aspects it is a powerful force. In the human organism the Blue Ray controls the Throat Chakram. The colour produces a calm, peaceful radiation and is excellent for all inflamed and feverish conditions.

THROAT DISEASES (e.g., Laryngitis)

Focus Blue Light on the throat for fifteen minutes at regular intervals. Give half a glass of blue-rayed water every half an hour. Blue Ray Breathing and meditation should be practised. The throat chakram is especially sensitive to mental currents.

SORE THROAT

The inflammation will quickly die down if blue-rayed water is used as a gargle at intervals of two or three hours. Focus Blue Light on the throat.

HOARSENESS

Small doses of blue-rayed water and exposure of the throat to Blue Light for thirty minutes.

Blue Ray Breathing and affirmation should be practised first thing in the morning.

GOITRE

Focus Blue Light on the throat for half an hour and administer magnetic massage. Gargle frequently with blue-charged water.

FEVERS

The application of Blue Light to the part inflamed by heat is beneficial and effective.

PALPITATION

Small doses of blue-rayed water alternatively with green-rayed water is an effective remedy.

BILIOUS ATTACKS

Blue-rayed water taken every hour is an effective treatment.

COLIC

The cooling blue-water vibration is a good remedy.
Allow one ounce every quarter of an hour.

JAUNDICE

Sitting regularly in a strong Blue Light is an effective aid in curing this disease. Small doses of blue-charged water also assist.

SKIN ABRASIONS, CUTS, BURNS, ETC.

The action of blue-rayed water lowers the burning vibration and reduces heat. The Blue Ray is an effective agent in stopping bleeding.

RHEUMATISM

The Blue Radiation is valuable in treating cases of acute Rheumatism. The chronic type of the disease is best combated by use of the Orange Ray.

THE INDIGO RAY

Indigo influences the central part of the head in the region of the pineal gland. The Ray exercises dominion over the eye, ear and nose. It is of great value in the treatment of certain forms of nervous and mental disorders. Its secondary use is in the treatment of lung diseases and Pneumonia, Asthma, Bronchitis, Consumption and Dyspepsia.

Indigo has a powerful influence on the mental and nervous organisation. It expels the negative elements in the consciousness and when rightly understood and applied is capable of building up and inducing higher and positive elements.

DEAFNESS

Concentrate Indigo Light on the defective ear or ears. This should be supplemented by Colour Breathing and by anointing the ears each morning with Indigo-charged water. The mental background of the complaint is important and may lead to an understanding of the cause. Deafness often owes its origin to wrong attitudes towards people in early life. Sufferers often lock themselves up in their subconscious mind, stifling the emotions instead of sublimating them. Any tendency to brooding, introversion and self-absorption must be checked.

CATARACT (Preliminary Treatment)

Indigo Breathing should first be practised and then the eyes should be bathed with Indigo-charged water ; wet flannels should be laid on the head and forehead for the preliminary treatment. In the second stage Indigo Rays are focused on the eye and its surrounding region for a period of thirty minutes and radiant magnetic massage is given. Attention should be paid to the psychological factors and by the visualisation of Rose-red beneficial effects will be experienced. (Second Treatment p. 80.)

DELIRIUM TREMENS

Use the Indigo Light on the head for fifteen to thirty minutes; supplement with small doses of Indigo-charged water.

EYE INFLAMMATION

This distressing condition is sometimes due to digestive disorders. In such cases the Blue and Indigo Rays are very helpful and the wearing of blue-coloured glasses will also assist. The face and head should be given Blue Light treatment. Ear diseases respond to careful treatment with Indigo Light, and Indigo-rayed water is also beneficial.

DYSPEPSIA

The effect of Blue Light and water is to increase the functioning of the digestive organs and to cleanse the system of the predisposing causes of the dyspeptic condition.

PNEUMONIA

The power of Indigo Light is very marked in cases of pneumonia. The light heals the cells of the lungs, lowers the temperature, reduces the feverishness and benefits the sufferer in various ways.

MENTAL DISORDERS

Good results have been obtained with Indigo Light in cases of insane excitability and violent tendencies. In cases of depression and debility, the Orange Ray is found effective.

The Violet Ray

The increasing use of Violet Rays in recent years is a striking testimony to the widespread belief in this form of treatment. Violet Ray treatment has become a popular practice, but it should not be used indiscriminately. Much harm can be done by improper and indiscriminate use of Violet Rays. It should be remembered that Violet is the the highest and most subtle specialisation of light and that this Ray corresponds with the highest elements in man's nature. Its main province is the brain and the mental and spiritual nature. It is not suited to minds that are undeveloped, retarded or stunted on account of its very high vibrational rate. It is the stimulator of the crown chakram and controls the pituitary gland.

Nervous Ailments

The Violet Ray acts very beneficially on the nervous system. It is especially beneficial for creative workers where nerves and mind are subject to much strain and stress. The opposite colour—affinity—Yellow—is excellent as an antidote to the periods of depression which often occur to highly-strung people. Colour-breathing is of great help in steadying the nerves and supplying fresh tone and vigour.

Insomnia

A great many people find the Violet Ray or its ancillary, the Amethyst Ray, a most effective way of overcoming sleeplessness. Some find it preferable to Blue or Indigo. Violet is best suited to the artistic temperament and to those with a great desire to express themselves on the creative plane of mind.

MENTAL DISORDERS

The use of soft Violet Light has been found of great benefit in the treatment of excitable cases. The Rays of the Blue group have a marked influence on the brain.

CATARACT

The experience of Dr. Babbitt and others testify to the good effect which Violet Rays exercise on the eyes and in overcoming optic disorders, including cataract.

Red is also a powerful curative agent. (See p. 77.)

CHAPTER 11

MENTAL AND ABSENT HEALING

IN the Cosmic System of Healing the use of Colour is combined with the force of Mind. The mental factor in health and disease is fully recognised. The true Colour Healer sees different levels of consciousness, such as the etheric, the mental, the causal and the spiritual, all of which contribute to in their final working out to the state of either harmony or disease in the physical.

The Colour Healer is aware that the infinite powers of Spirit manifesting in the White Light flow into each individual through the magnetic Aura. In the degree to which the Aura reciprocates to the divine inflow, so personal harmony and well-being is the result. In the case of the spiritual, emotional or etheric maladjustments appearing in the personality in various forms such as emotional and nervous tension, feelings of bitterness, resentment, frustration, hatred and the mental complexes of fear, worry, inferiority, selfishness, etc., the divine inflow of Love, Health and Harmony does not reach the centre of man's being. It is stopped through wrong thinking or the wrong vibration or wrong action, with the result that a blank area, so to speak, is formed, which swiftly becomes the breeding-ground of negative, evil or undivine thoughts and elements which work themselves out as diseased conditions of all kinds.

Just as the root or plant that cannot catch the sunlight becomes a stunted, faded, undeveloped organism, so the individual who is cut off from the White Light of the

Spirit becomes ill and defective, a victim of his own false or perverted mind.

The main characteristic of true mind or intelligence is responsiveness, recognition, and the whole action of the Universal or Cosmic Mind in bringing the evolutionary process from its first beginnings to its present human stage is achieved by a continual intelligent response which the demand which each stage in the progress has made for an adjustment between itself and its environment.

The Colour-healer recognises a universal intelligence permeating all things and also sees a corresponding responsiveness hidden deep down in their nature and ready to be called into action when appealed to.

Colour Treatment is based on the principle that all healing is a change of mental attitude or belief. The subconscious or subjective mind is the creative faculty within us and creates whatever the conscious mind impresses upon it. The conscious mind, the vehicle of the intellect, impresses its thoughts and ideas upon it which are the expression of the belief. Thus the creation of the subconscious self is the manifestation of our beliefs.

The primary aim of healing is to change the wrong consciousness and beliefs. Very frequently the wrong state of consciousness which externalises as illness or disease is the mistaken idea that some secondary cause which is really only a condition is the primary cause.

In reality there is only one primary cause for such phenomena, viz.: the subjective or subconscious mind. The subconscious mind is so primitive, basic, and elemental, with roots so deep in our being, that its power is difficult to comprehend. It belongs to the plane of the absolute, it functions without the limitations of time and space, whereas the conscious mind or intellect perceives things in the limited aspect of form and time and space.

If you ever conceive of yourself in the absolute or unconditioned the conception that arises is that of pure living spirit, unhampered by conditions of any kind and therefore not subject to illness. This mental concept must be impressed upon the subconscious mind of the patient being treated and it will become externalised.

It is not always easy to apply this principle in practice because most people have held all their lives the false belief that disease is a substantial entity, a reality in itself, and is of course looked upon as a primary cause instead of as a merely negative condition resulting from the *absence* of a primary cause. It is a common occurrence in healing that after a definite improvement in the patient's health has become apparent the old symptoms reappear. This is because the new belief in his own creative faculty and in the power of Colour has not fully penetrated into the subconscious. Each succeeding treatment and each application of Colour-rays helps the subconscious mind to build up the right attitude until finally the permanent cure is effected.

In the mental aspect of healing the Healer substitutes his own conscious mind and will for that of the patient in order to reach the patient's subconscious mind and to impress upon it the conception of perfect health. The Healer likewise impresses upon the subconscious mind of the patient certain colours which he knows will give the right healing vibration.

A question that will be asked is—" How can the Healer substitute his own conscious mind for that of the patient ?" The patient is asked to put himself in a receptive mental attitude which is not the same thing as blacking out his mind or surrendering his will. He is asked to exercise his will so as to remove the barrier of his own objective personality and to open his mind to the thought-force of the Healer. The Healer adopts the same attitude but in a reverse manner : while the patient lays aside the personality barrier with the object of allowing the power to flow in, the Healer does so with the object of allowing the power to flow out.

True healing is a partnership between healer and patient. The mutual removal of the personality barrier results in the condition known as contact or rapport—the cosmic forces will then be polarised according to the universal law of Nature. The finer forces of light and colour operate best when harmony exists. When the personality barriers which are similar to the language barriers between persons of different nationality have been removed the Healer can address the subconscious self of the patient as though it were his own. If we concentrate the mind on the diseased condition of the patient we are conscious of him as a separate personality which is the antithesis of pure spirit. The right attitude is the conception of him as a ray of pure spirit which enables us to contact his innermost being.

The Colour-healer withdraws his thought from the contemplation of symptoms and from the physical-personality aspect and thinks of him as a spiritual being composed of pure light, not subject to any conditions and able to externalise all the spiritual qualities inherent within.

With this concept firmly held in his mind the Healer can then make mental affirmations that he shall build up in the physical and etheric bodies the correspondence of that spiritual vitality which exists deep within. This thought-form is moulded by the Healer's conscious mind at the same time that the patient's conscious mind is accepting or believing the fact that he is receiving the thought-stream of the Healer. As a result of this mental process the patient's subconscious mind becomes firmly impressed with the recognition of its own vital and health-giving power. The subconscious mind, aided by the restorative vibrations of Colour, carries into outward manifestation the picture impressed upon it : the negative condition of illness then gives way to new health.

It will be seen in the above statement that no attempt is made to dominate or hypnotise the patient's mind. The aim is to arouse and strengthen the patient's own resources by a partnership of harmony and co-operation. To achieve this mental partnership it is very necessary to instruct the patient in the broad principles of spiritual Colour-healing. Sometimes, however, this may not be possible or advisable. Patients may have deeply-rooted prejudices, scepticism, resentment or extreme detachment which make conscious and voluntary rapport impossible. The alternative method, that of Absent-healing, may then be applied.

Since the healing rays are universal and omnipresent and the subconscious mind or the higher consciousness is not limited in its power of action to the senses or the dimension of time and space, it is therefore quite imma-terial whether the patient be in the immediate presence of the Healer or in a distant country.

The essence of Absent Colour Treatments is the holding in the mind a Colour that is required for healing the sufferer. At some previously agreed-on time the Healer should enter his Sanctuary of Colour or take his place before a Colour Shrine or Altar dedicated to the trans-mission of the Rays and then tune-in mentally with the correct Colour Ray. He should hold the letter of the patient and impress upon his mind the name and address : this should be repeated several times. He then reviews rapidly in his mind the symptoms or the disease to be treated and afterwards concentrates on the following (or some similar) formula : " I project to so-and-so the Orange Ray of vitality and restoration and call upon the Cosmic Power to aid me in this work of restoring health and harmony to his system. Through the White Light of Spirit I call forth the latent powers within his being to cast out the negative conditions of disease. I direct the Cosmic Healing Rays to replenish his Aura and remove all roots and causes of his disease." He repeats the patient's name again and at the same time radiates from his Aura whatever colours he desires to send out.

It is not necessary to devote any great length of time to each individual patient : from three to five minutes expended on each is usually sufficient. The patient for his part should remain passive and receptive for about one hour so that his depleted system may fully absorb the cosmic healing vibrations.

Although this Colour Treatment is purely on the mental-spiritual plane it is helpful in some cases to turn on a Colour-lamp during the treatment period. This uplifts the physical vibrations and creates a fitting atmosphere. The patient should be advised as to the time of the treatment and should be asked to hold himself in a relaxed and receptive state of mind. This is not to say that healers cannot do good to sufferers without their knowledge—this is being done every day. The Healing Rays are well able to benefit a patient without his knowledge or expectation just as a thought can be impressed on the minds of most people at any time by telepathy. But it is found in practice that the conscious co-operation of healer and patient is the best arrangement in Absent Treatments.

A word may here be said about the value of sending healing vibrations at night. If you are in pain or trouble yourself, such a thought-radiation sent to a friend will lighten your pain or worry : if you are sleepless, it will swiftly tranquillise your mind, restoring the nerve-balance and flooding your system with harmony : if you awake during the night you will quickly regain rest by recalling the suffering of some patient and sending out a healing vibration.

An important link between healer and patient is the writing of letters. A letter conveys far more than the written sentences it contains—it carries the vital magnetism and radiations of the writer, including the thought-aura. The patient should be encouraged to write periodically concerning his health condition and the Healer should answer him promptly. A personal letter, not a duplicated circular, should always be sent.

Finally, the student of Colour-healing should bear in mind the words of a great spiritual master : " A mental Colour Treatment is an activity of great beauty and power in the higher planes and is of great benefit and refreshment to the Healer as well as to the patient."

UNIVERSAL AFFIRMATION

" I am surrounded at all times by Cosmic Healing Rays and I wish to become fully receptive to them."

This statement should be affirmed several times daily until the student becomes really Ray-conscious. The Cosmic student uses mental affirmations for all Colour Practice and Healing.

HOW TO USE THE COLOUR RAYS

One of the best ways to receive the blessings and benefits of the Colour Vibrations is to use a suitable electric Colour Lamp specially made for the purpose.

COLOUR PRACTICE

1. To Obtain Health, Vitality and Pure Blood

Use the Rose-red and Orange Rays. They are rich in vitality-globules, the essence of Prana. Red, being the blood colour, is easily visualised and it is easy to affirm mentally that the Rose current is flowing through your blood-stream.

The consciousness of pure blood is a great aid in maintaining good health. Orange—the Vitality Ray—is another colour you should picture as surrounding and permeating every cell in your body.

2. For Re-Building the Health After Illness

Tune yourself to the Green, Blue, and Violet Rays. Change your thoughts if they are grey, dull or colourless, to bright, cheerful radiant thoughts of ease, health and peace. Health will come if you will throw away your mental blinds and let the colours in ! Affirm repeatedly the thought of Health as you draw in your Rays and you will effect a surprising change in yourself.

3. For Depression, Loneliness, Frustration, etc.

If you are feeling depressed and lonely let your mind vibrate to all the Seven Rays. The more you think of the inexhaustible Colour Forces surrounding you, the less lonely and despondent you will be. Your despondency and depression will disappear like grey clouds before the sunshine. The Cosmic teachings by their inherent fullness and their inspiring and stimulating qualities will absorb your thoughts and will release you from the vibrations that have been holding you down.

Clear Golden Yellow is one of the most powerful forces against depression and limitations of every kind.

4. FOR PROSPERITY, SUCCESS, PROGRESS, ETC.

Are your material sources limited ? Are you a victim of poverty-vibrations ? The Cosmic remedy is the Green Ray—the great source of Universal Supply. This vibration will attract the things you want. It is the Colour that enriches the personality and raises the vibrations of success and plenty. Affirm that you are tuned-in to the Green Ray of Supply and that you wish to demonstrate its power.

5. FOR MENTAL DEVELOPMENT, MIND POWER, ETC.

The way to attain the greater mental efficiency is to harmonise with the Golden Ray of Mind. This powerful ray emanates from the Infinite Centre of Wisdom and, by continual concentration, you will become in harmony with it. Whenever you find yourself in a dark passage in life turn to the Golden Cosmic Ray for light and illumination.

Seven Rules for Health and the Mastery of Negative Conditions

1. Bar from your mind the thought-forms of illness, trouble, worry, fear and all limitations.

2. Remember always that negative conditions begin by wrong-thinking.

3. Thoughts are vital and creative—therefore, *think* good and true things for yourself.

4. Visualise yourself in a peaceful state of health and happiness surrounded by the Seven Eternal Rays.

5. Practise your selected affirmation with a set mind and will.

6. In using the Colour Lamp or Chart consciously realise that you are receiving your supply of Cosmic Force.

7. Cultivate your self-reliance and do not allow others to influence you against your better judgment.

NOTES ON THE COLOUR RAYS

(For a full analysis and description of the Cosmic Colour Rays the reader is referred to the Preliminary Course of the C.C.F.)

1. Concentrate for 10–20 minutes on each colour in turn —one colour daily for a week.

2. The Colour Rays are representatives of the Cosmic Lights—realise that they are spiritual forces perpetually flowing towards and through you.

3. The Colours work through the glandular centres of the body. The principle behind Colour Healing is the regulation of the flow of the Colour forces by consciously absorbing them as needed, using each Ray with the specific purpose of rebuilding and revitalising every organ of the body *through the etheric counterpart.*

4. Regular and systematic practice will gradually transform your body, mind and spirit. The general health will improve, the mind will become more efficient, and the spirit-self more sensitive and developed.

5. The Colour method soon becomes a *sub-conscious* function ; Colour being one of the fundamental

elements in the universe, acts on the subconscious mind which is an important source of health and vitality, whilst life in general assumes a happier outlook.

PRACTICAL PROCEDURE

If you possess a room set aside for Colour Culture the exercises should be performed there. Failing this, we recommend that a corner of your private room be set aside as a Colour Sanctuary. It is a great advantage to have some place consecrated to Colour as it will increase the flow of vibrations and will soon develop into a Cosmic power-station.

Before commencing the exercises, start with Colour Breathing as given in Lesson 1 of the Preliminary Course.

Take a sitting position with the spine erect and the hands folded across the chest just over the solar plexus. The Chart should be hung on the wall opposite your chair and as near as possible on a level with your eyes.

For general training in Colour work on the following system :—

1. ROSE-RED. (Stimulating and Uplifting) After concentrating for three minutes on the Rose-red colour turn to gaze inwards to the solar plexus and affirm mentally — " The Rose-red Cosmic Ray is flowing through my blood-stream, eliminating the poisons and giving me new vitality and vigour." Repeat seven times, visualising the Colour with your eyes closed. When you have drawn in the Ray you will be

conscious of a pleasant glow spreading through the whole body. It is excellent for tiredness, depression and depletion.

2. ORANGE (Stimulating and Re-vitalising)

This is the basic health colour. Meditate on this bright, cheering colour for three minutes or until you can visualise it clearly. Then silently affirm—" The Orange Ray is flowing through my glands, invigorating and re-vitalising them." Repeat seven times. The Orange Ray is a powerful tonic for all conditions of nervous exhaustion.

3. GREEN (Sedative, Relaxant, Rhythmic)

Concentrate on this radiant colour until you feel you are vibrating in harmony with it ; then affirm—" The Green Cosmic Ray is flowing through my heart and nervous system, restoring rhythm and strength to my nerves." Repeat seven times. This colour is excellent for nervous strain and anxiety-conditions—it gives a delightful sense of peace and restfulness.

The above three Colours act specifically on the physical, etheric and emotional nature. They govern all our material needs—health, vitality, love, prosperity, well-being, etc.

4. BLUE (Electric, Cooling, Soothing)

Meditate on this beautiful colour until you feel you are drawing the vibrations into your innermost being. This Ray belongs to the Ethereal and Spiritual group and you should be conscious of a vibrational feeling somewhat different from the three preceding colours. Affirm—" The Blue Cosmic Ray is flowing into and through my physical tissues removing the poisons from them and re-vitalising them." Repeat seven times. The Blue Ray is very useful for sore throat, laryngitis, feverish conditions and eye-troubles.

5. YELLOW (Stimulating, Illuminating)

Concentrate on this luminous colour and visualise it flooding your brain with its golden light. Then affirm—" I am vibrating to the Yellow Cosmic Ray and drawing it into my solar plexus. My brain, spinal cord, and nerves are being stimulated and energised." Repeat seven times. This Ray has a healing effect on digestive troubles, stomach disorders and complaints of the circulatory system.

6. VIOLET (Stimulating, Purifying)

Meditate on this spiritual colour until you feel it flowing through your body, cleaning away everything that is harmful. Then affirm—" The Violet Ray is flowing into my pineal gland and is healing and re-vitalising every part of my being." Repeat seven times. This Ray acts on the head-glands, curing headaches, insomnia, neuralgia and inflammation of the nerves.

7. The WHITE   The Colour Treatment is concluded
   LIGHT   by affirming—" The White Light of
   (Universal   Universal Spiritual Healing is filling
   Regenera-   my whole being with Cosmic Energy,
   tive)   health and peaceful vibrations.

CHAPTER 12

RADIANT HEALERS

By M. MacKay, reprinted from *Radiance Magazine*

Colour is a powerful Cosmic Force. Its value as a healing Agent is now widely recognised. Mr. MacKay, who is a world-travelled lecturer, explains how the Cosmic Rays can be applied to the healing of the body by mental concentration. The Author

In these days of darkness with all the prevailing miseries I would point a way out, for I fully believe I can do so. In remote places of the world, in the midst of many and varied dangers, I was far from help or advice from any European doctor. I did not despair in these trying conditions, for I was always comforted by the fact that I had ever at my beck and call an amazing storehouse—a natural laboratory and dispensary combined.

The help I needed for myself and the faithful coloured people who accompanied ·me into the hinterland of Central Africa came from my Seven Healers. Let me introduce them to you. My first healer is a Soother of Pain. These Healers, by the way, are not persons, nevertheless they are very real Healers in times of sickness.

BLUE

The Pain Healer is the Blue Cosmic Ray

This powerful Healing Ray will definitely help you to banish your own pain and also that of your friends. Whether they are absent or present will not make the

95

slightest difference. I would like you to put this Blue— Sapphire Blue Ray—to the test. These Cosmic Rays are always beaming forth, earthwards. Cold and foggy days can never prevent the fulfilment of their life-sustaining purpose.

If you have an acute pain, repeat the following affirmation seven times :—" The powerful Sapphire Blue Cosmic Ray is permeating my body, soul and spirit, giving me perfect health."

Visualise this mighty Blue Ray as entering your body via your solar plexus. If you should be the victim of Insomnia the following remedy will enable you to escape from this nerve-depressing malady. First concentrate on the colour known as Cobalt Blue. Then make this sevenfold affirmation :—" I am now contacting the *Cobalt Blue Ray*. Under its beauteous influence I fully relax. I enjoy sweet peace, and nights of joyous health-giving sleep, undisturbed and pure." It is most advisable that the Cobalt Blue be clearly visualised. The affirmation is to be used when the patient is settled comfortably in bed.

INDIGO

The Cosmic Ray of Inner Knowledge and Wisdom

Students and those in pursuit of Knowledge will be greatly helped by visualising the Ray of Indigo Blue. This produces a receptivity of mind, which is most helpful to students of all classes. It is equally efficacious in Psychic and Spiritual Studies. Use this affirmation seven times. " I now contact the Indigo Blue Ray. Under its influence I receive that Knowledge so beneficial to me."

There is also another wonderful Medical Ray which, if only known, would often be contacted by healers of all classes. I have visualised this Ray on several occasions during actual healing. It is *White Flecked Pale Blue*. I am positive that all healers work in varied degrees to the influx of this Ray. To invoke its aid by the sevenfold repeated affirmation will be most beneficial to Healer and Patient. " I am now contacting the *White Flecked Pale Blue Ray*. Through its powerful influence, Healing and Peace are outpoured."

ROSE-RED

The Ray of Universal Love Life and Vitality

It may be that you are anaemic or know of some friend who would welcome the Healing of this distressing malady, which will follow the opening up of their receptive being to the mighty *Rose-Red Ray* with the help of the following affirmation repeated seven times :—" The Rose-Red Cosmic Ray is flowing through my blood stream, giving me an abundant supply of rich, healthy red blood."

GREEN

The Ray of Balance Harmony and Abundance

There are thousands of people who are irritable and depressed, troubled with nervous disorders in varying degrees. Every one of these can be greatly helped by accepting the guidance herein offered and will see a vast improvement in their health and nerves in a short space of time. These people should open up their receptive being via the solar plexus and use the following affirmation, seven times repeated :—" The soothing Emerald Green Ray of the mighty Cosmos is permeating my being with peace, rest and contentment, and giving me the fullest confidence that all my needs both material and spiritual are supplied by the Holy Spirit through His Universal Attributes."

YELLOW

The Ray of the Cosmic Sun and The Christos

The *Yellow Cosmic Ray* is a great Spiritual Ray. Visualise this as a Golden Ray entering your body via the solar plexus whilst you affirm seven times the following :—

" The *Golden Yellow Cosmic Ray* is permeating my body, soul and spirit with the Divine Love and Wisdom of God. As I receive this God-gift I vow to dedicate its uses to those who may be in need of it, both materially and spiritually." This Ray is also termed The Ray of Sight. It gives both physical (external) and Clairvoyance (inner) vision.

ORANGE

The Cosmic Ray of Etheric Vitality and Energy

Should your trouble be loss of vitality and listlessness then you are in need of the restoring Orange Ray and should repeat the following seven times :—" The Life-giving Orange Ray of the Cosmos permeates my being by way of the solar plexus filling me with vitality and the joy of life, revivifying my glands, re-charging my etheric body, and rejuvenating every atom and particle of my being."

VIOLET

The Ray of Mysticism

This Cosmic Ray is helpful to all who would develop the Inner Mind. By its power much that has hitherto been understood but vaguely is transmuted into a concrete reality. The Soul is revealed in its pristine purity and the student becomes the Knower. The Violet Ray is also known as the *Voice of God*. When the student recognises this voice he is fully illumined.

RED

The Ray Ruling Every Form of Life

If you possess a goodly measure of health and healing power it is good that you should continue so. You will be continually benefited in this purpose by using the following affirmation seven times repeated :—" The Red Cosmic Ray is permeating my being with radiant health, strength, and the zest of life."

Remember that if you practise deep breathing as you make your affirmations the power is increased.

By M. MACDONALD-BAYNE

The Higher Power You Can Use

These lessons were previously only given privately but now the course has been put into book form so that all may embrace this Higher Power for immediate use and benefit in their lives.

Through the super-technique explained in this course there comes a supreme understanding, it goes beyond all psychological and mind training methods, it supersedes Yoga exercises and lifts you into a realm where this Intelligent Power becomes active in your life without effort.

"I am the Life"

This is a sequel to *The Higher Power You Can Use* which will fulfil the great longing of those who desire to know the deepest inner truths of life and the realisation of their highest riches by unfolding the mighty Power within, enabling the reader to solve all personal problems gaining complete freedom under all circumstances, thus assuring a healthy and happy life.

It gives in simple language the mighty word of power and the teaching of Jesus is portrayed in simple and clear statements.

By M. MACDONALD-BAYNE

Heal Yourself

Think what would be yours if the Laws of Life revealed in this book had been given to you long ago! You would have been carried forward from Victory to Victory, sickness would have disappeared and Health would have been established.

Do not wait another moment—but make yourself acquainted with them and you will find the shortest way to Health and Happiness, not only for yourself but for others too.

Spiritual and Mental Healing

The greatest service given to humanity is curing the afflictions of mind and body and there is still hope for those who have been abandoned when they learn to put themselves in conscious union with the healing power of the Universe and apply the Spiritual, Mental and Natural Laws scientifically.

So-called chronic and incurable conditions have been effectively and permanently cured by the application of the knowledge that is revealed.

The most modern scientific knowledge combined with the wisdom of the Masters is the foundation of this magnificent work.

By M. MACDONALD-BAYNE

What is Mine is Thine
How to Use Your Divine Power
(*In Two Volumes*)

These two volumes reveal the inner secrets of our Divine Power over disease, want and confusion, and will tell you how to apply this knowledge and power for all practical purposes to acquire health, happiness and success in life.

Each lecture is followed by a short item for meditation and consists of a simple exposition of great spiritual truths, couched in language which is acceptable to the layman, as Christian phraseology is used.

How to Relax and Re-vitalize Yourself

You can make yourself a real creative personality among men and women of the world by following the instructions given in this remarkable book. Everyone needs these instructions, for it has been proved that almost 100 per cent of sickness, mental, physical and unsuccessful living is caused by Tension in one way or another.

Written in easy understandable language this scientific and self-reorganising knowledge has been made available to all and will be a treasure to anyone who will carry out the practical and essential instructions so necessary in this fast moving age of ours.

By M. MACDONALD-BAYNE

Divine Healing of Mind and Body

(The Master Speaks Again)

The story behind the compilation of this work is one of the most thrilling and inspiring dramas of our present age. It was not written in the ordinary way but was recorded as spoken in flawless language, and the words recorded reveal an influence beyond the mind of man which will satisfy the consuming desire of those who want to solve the mystery of life and the healing of mind and body.

The wisdom of the ancients will inspire all who read this book and give them that assurance which will lift the thinking of man into a realm of understanding and freedom thereby eliminating fear.